PRAISE

Dr. Susie Gronski's book *Pelvic Pain: The U...*
read if you suffer from pelvic pain or hav... ....
like the way she talks when treating people, her communication style is
down to earth and she makes sure you 'get it.' And she really knows her
shit! Above all, her message is one of hope and resilience. Buy this book!

STEVE JELLERSON
Staunton, VA

In a factual yet humorous way, Dr. Susie Gronski's *Pelvic Pain: The
Ultimate Cock Block* provides both answers and solutions towards re-
gaining your manpower. Covering all bases, she perfectly pitches all
you need to know about male anatomy, pain science, brain training,
sexual function, exercise and treatment options. Written in a language
style that every man and his partner will relate to, I cannot more highly
recommend this text. So, if you've got a spare hour or two, be kind to
yourself! You'll find there's a toolbox of skills to help regain your pride
and your passion… and an end to the 'cock block' in your jocks! Hey—
it may just be the best investment you'll ever make! Prost!

JO MILIOS, men's health physiotherapist, Western Australia
www.menshealthphysiotherapy.com.au

Pelvic Pain: The Ultimate Cock Block by Dr. Susie Gronski is an expertly
written book on male pelvic pain conditions, including chronic pelvic
pain syndrome (CPPS) and chronic prostatitis (CP). It is a must-read for
patients (and their partners) wanting to take control of their symptoms
and their recovery. This honest and open guide offers a window into
Susie's highly reputable approach to male pelvic pain, balancing hard
science, humour and very practical, easy-to-implement self-care techniques. This beautifully illustrated upfront self-help guide is *the* book for
patients who wish to be the driver in their recovery, not just a passenger.

KARL MONAHAN, founder of The Pelvic Pain Clinic in London,
a clinic solely dedicated to the treatment of male pelvic pain conditions
www.thepelvicpainclinic.co.uk

Dr. Susie Gronski, a gifted physical therapist, has written a ground-breaking book on male pelvic pain. *Pelvic Pain: The Ultimate Cock Block* is a user-friendly guide that helps men understand why they have pain and what to do about it. Male pelvic pain is a forgotten piece of our healthcare puzzle, and Dr. Gronski brings it back to life in an easy-to-read manual that every man experiencing pelvic pain should have on his bookshelf. I really enjoyed Dr. Gronski's writing style, and the exercises with illustrations presented are so easy to follow. If you're a guy suffering from pelvic pain, don't hesitate to pick up a copy and begin your journey to becoming pain-free!

Dr. Nikolas Hedberg, author of
The Complete Thyroid Health & Diet Guide
www.drhedberg.com

After far too many excruciating months of pain and discomfort in my nether regions and no answers (but plenty of unnecessary pain and frustration from the traditional group of medical specialists), I feel blessed to have found Dr. Susie Gronski on the internet. She literally saved my life as she guided me on a path to heal myself from pelvic pain. Dr. Susie is nothing short of amazing! She has what most doctors today sorely lack... great compassion, accessibility, knowledge, humor, and gentle care for her patients. Dr. Susie Gronski is the real deal! Run, don't walk to her special approach to healing. She is the gold standard for doctor-patient care!

Bruce Lecure
Professor Emeritus, University of Miami

Dr. Susie Gronski's book *Pelvic Pain: The Ultimate Cock Block* is a must-read for any man experiencing pelvic pain. It is well-written, insightful and full of practical advice. For those men who have been baffled by what's going on down below, this book goes a long way in helping to normalize the experience. We're not nuts after all! Thanks, Dr. G!

Dan P., Glen Mills, PA

Thank you, Susie, for all of your hard work putting this hilariously helpful resource together and striving to make sure it contains the best, most up-to-date evidence. This book is a brilliant resource for anyone who has ever had pain, with a few frank and beans jokes thrown in for fun.

KATELYN FRITZ, PT, MPT

I'm a male in my late 50's who began experiencing an ache in what felt like the bottom of my being which intensified after sexual activity. Over about eight months, it worsened. Neither my MD nor a urologist had any specific ideas for relief. I suffered physically and doubted my viability going forward until I got a newsletter from my doctor introducing me to Dr. Susie's practice.

It would be difficult to overstate how helpful Dr. Susie was from the time I made contact with her to after only our third session. By that time, the ache had largely disappeared, and I was able to be sexually active without pain. I now have techniques and a way of understanding and managing so the ache is either non-existent or a relatively minor and temporary inconvenience.

I highly recommend seeing Dr. Susie for any and all male issues in the nether regions.

ANONYMOUS, USA

PELVIC PAIN

THE ULTIMATE COCK BLOCK

A no-bullshit guide for men navigating through pelvic pain

SUSIE GRONSKI, PT, DPT

First published in 2017
Second edition 2020
Copyright © 2017, 2020 by Susie Gronski

Cover design and typesetting by Stewart A. Williams
Interior illustrations by Weronika Zubek at TwoEasels
Front cover photo: © Juan Moyano / Stocksy United

Dr. Susie Gronski, Inc.
56 Central Avenue, Suite 103
Asheville, NC 28801
drsusieg.com

Printed in the United States of America

Library of Congress Cataloging-in-Publication data
Library of Congress Control Number: 2020909308

Gronski, Susie, 1985-
Pelvic Pain The Ultimate Cock Block: A no-bullshit guide for men navigating through pelvic pain / Susie Gronski
cm.
Includes bibliographical references
ISBN 978-0-9986957-2-3 (paperback)
ISBN 978-0-9986957-3-0 (e-book)
ISBN 978-0-9986957-4-7 (audio)

DISCLAIMER
This information is provided for educational and informational purposes only. It is provided to educate you about *pelvic health and wellness* as a self-help tool for your own use. It is not intended *to be a substitute for professional diagnosis or treatment.* This information is to be used at your own risk, based on your own judgment. For the author's full disclaimer, please go to drsusieg.com/disclaimer.

AFFILIATE DISCLOSURE
From time to time, the author may promote, affiliate with, or partner with other individuals or businesses whose programs, products and services align with her own. The author is highly selective and only promotes partners whose programs, products and/or services she respects. In the spirit of transparency, please be aware that there may be instances when this book promotes, markets, shares or sells programs, products or services for other partners and in exchange the author may receive financial compensation or other rewards. For the author's full affiliate disclosure, please go to drsusieg.com/disclaimer.

DEDICATION

For the men who have been told they 'just have to live with it' for the rest of their lives.

FOREWORD

In 2016, I had never heard of pelvic floor physical therapy. Like many guys, perhaps most, my limited discussions about male pelvic pain or prostate issues came from cringeworthy stories, jokes, or very brief descriptions of someone else's cancer surgery. So, when my urologist told me a pelvic floor physical therapist (PFPT) might be able to help me recover after my second prostate surgery in three weeks, my response was equal parts confusion and skepticism. The urologist gave me a couple of recommendations, but suggested I do some research to find out more about what was involved. That research opened my eyes to an incredible service gap for men suffering from pelvic pain and eventually led me to Dr. Susie Gronski.

I live in Houston, fourth-largest city in the US, home to a booming economy and world-renowned medical center with experts of every kind. If you had asked me if I thought I would have trouble finding a physical therapist nearby, I would have told you there are probably more physical therapists within a five-mile radius of my home than there are restaurants. And there are restaurants everywhere. I assumed finding a PFPT would be easy. I was wrong.

What I found was that – in Houston, at least – most men who are referred to PFPTs are referred after prostate removal, usually due to cancer, and those physical therapy treatments are typically short-term. The primary goal is usually to help regain continence. One physical therapist told me she typically only needs one or two sessions to treat her patients and never needs to do an exam. She just talks them through a Kegel or two, and they're happy to be finished with the process. The fact that I didn't have cancer but was still being referred for treatment was clearly confusing to her. She said she had never had a patient like that before.

Along the way, I talked with another physical therapist who had recently moved out of the Houston area. She resonated with the lack of men's pelvic health awareness and practitioners not only in Houston but nationwide. She was the one who recommended I read this book. "It has a rather provocative title," she said with a chuckle, "so it should be easy to find." She described Dr. Gronski as "a wonderful human being," and said the book was an excellent resource for treating pelvic pain. I ordered the book immediately, read it, and agreed with her assessment on both counts. The book is packed with information, but is, at the same time, funny and straightforward, practical and direct. As I read, I felt like I finally had some hope and was beginning to understand the 'why' behind my pelvic pain.

Eventually, I found a PFPT in Houston and began treatments, but my situation was complicated. In the end, I had a total of three prostate surgeries and a hip surgery within a 10-month period. My doctors were proficient and caring, but they were still recommending three more surgeries to address the ongoing pain and spasms I was experiencing.

Desperate for an alternative to more surgeries, I made my way to Asheville, 1,000 miles from Houston, for a six-day intensive with Dr. Susie. That trip was life-changing. She is, in person, what you would expect from reading her book. Knowledgeable, skilled, funny, compassionate. She not only gave me hope, but I left Asheville pain-free for the first time in more than a year. Dr. Susie taught me how to know what my brain was and wasn't telling me when I experienced pain and how to reframe the way I responded to my body's protective alerts. I returned to Houston armed with the tools I needed to recover and was able to avoid surgeries five, six, and seven.

Dr. Gronski's work is paving the way for men to have the freedom and the space to talk about their pelvic health struggles without pretense, judgment, or shame. Whether you are reading this book at the beginning of your journey or looking for help because it seems like no one else is listening, you are in the right place. This book helps demystify pelvic pain and provides real solutions for treatment and recovery. I, for one, am immensely grateful to have found it and its author, Dr. Susie G.

Steve Johnson
Houston, TX

CONTENTS

INTRODUCTION

You woke up one morning expecting a hard-on, but instead all you felt was dick pain. You thought maybe it was a weird sex position or that sports injury from the other day. *No biggie, it'll go away,* you told yourself. Or maybe you had no clue how it happened but you were sure it would sort itself out eventually.

Now you're not so sure...

Years later, you're still dealing with the same nightmare and have no answers. You've tried everything but the medications haven't worked, and the doctors don't know what else to do. Your penis just doesn't work the same anymore. You think about it all the time, freaked out that there's something else more serious going on that the docs just haven't found yet.

Did I hit the nail on the head?

Who am I to help?

You're probably thinking to yourself, *But you're a chick. What do you know about having penis pain?* And you're right. I don't have a penis. But here's a knowledge nugget for you... Even though our private parts look and are organized differently, they still work in a similar way.

To be honest, as a licensed doctor of physical therapy, certified pelvic rehabilitation practitioner, and long-time teacher of health programs that help men with pelvic pain become experts in treating themselves, I'm simply fed up with the lack of care that guys get going the traditional medical route. I've seen too many of you walk into my office – indeed, people reaching out from all over the globe, from Europe to Australia, Asia to South America – complaining of pelvic pain that's been wreaking havoc in your life for years. It's not necessary.

Why this book?

A United States national survey from 1990 to 1994 reported that nearly two million outpatient visits per year were due to 'prostatitis' related issues.[1] Unfortunately, this label can include everything under the sun and is most likely used as an umbrella diagnosis to cover a myriad of symptoms. (And for insurance billing purposes, gotta code something to get paid.) There's definitely no shortage of men asking for help and, sadly, many are turned away when tests and scans come back negative. (Gulp. *Now what?!*)

Oftentimes, healthcare providers, through no fault of their own, are unaware or lack understanding about how pain works. Believe it or not, there's relatively little contemporary pain science education in the medical community across all professions. Indeed, this knowledge has been around for decades, but conventional treatment remains vested in a purely biomedical model. This stuff is not taught in schools either, but it definitely should be and is slowly making its way into the classroom.[2] Some are afraid to tackle these symptoms because they don't know what to do other than prescribe you antibiotics, anti-inflammatories, alpha-blockers, antidepressants or pain medications (all of which do have a time and a place and can be helpful when appropriate). As I said, it's not their fault that they take this approach; they're just trying to help you with the tools (and time) they have in their toolbox and within their institutions. More broadly, I see a lack of safe space for men, somewhere they can feel heard and understood, which is a complicating factor. This, coupled with distrust of the medical community because of dismissive and negative healthcare visits, leads many men to feel they have nowhere left to turn.

Hearing a medical professional say "There's nothing else I can do for you" might feel like a death sentence. Then there's all the googling that you've probably done about your symptoms. Let me guess. You're feeling straight up bummed and hopeless, like there's no cure. So, you're just going to have to get used to living this way, right? Wrong! It's not 'all in your head.' And no, you don't have to live with it for the rest of your life.

You've got to know all your options and become the expert in your own health. That's why I've written this book so that guys like you can realize pelvic pain isn't permanent, so that you know those options and so that you can better care for yourself down there. You can have your life back, and I'm going to show you how.

Why the updated edition?

If you're already familiar with my work from the first edition of *Pelvic Pain: The Ultimate Cock Block*, you might be wondering what's changed since my fingers hit the keyboard in 2015. And in my practice, the answer is a lot. I have been on a quest for knowledge and understanding of the psychological impacts and sociocultural influences of pain on someone's life. I am dedicated to adapting my practice to the latest in pain science, men's sexual health and pelvic health.

And so, as I navigate this world and work with more and more people, I expand my view and my outlook. I have come to realize that the most meaningful, impactful ways I can help someone is to help them transform *their own situation* to get their life back. As my experiences, knowledge and understanding of some complex topics deepen, my approach and practical advice encompass that as well.

My practice has evolved. So, too, must this book. The main reason for this updated edition is to keep the research in it as current as possible, because I am constantly learning and adapting to the knowledge and the evidence that's being presented as we come to learn more and more about how pain works. In addition to the biological underpinnings of pain, this edition is more psychologically informed and has a reflective style. This update is written to empower you and to take you on a self-guided discovery.

So, what's new?

Pain is very complex. That's not new. But what we know about it is always updating. What's new in this edition is a whole bunch of recent pain science. The more I learn about pain and the psychological, biological and sociocultural influences on pain, the more I see a well-rounded picture of health.

In this edition, you'll find out more on:

> ➤ why some common assumptions about pain are completely false

➤ how the nerves, the gut and the immune system come into play
➤ what causes suffering and how to shift your perspective
➤ how simple mindful practices and breathing can modulate pain
➤ how exploring your relationship with your pain is key to feeling better.

The bottom line of what you're about to find out in this book is this: Pain is personal. How you feel about it matters. And that's very good news when it comes to taking back control of your journey, knowing you can navigate your way through it and that there is hope for your pain to change.

Making the most of this book

Pelvic Pain: The Ultimate Cock Block has been written as a resource guide. You can read all the way through to understand the whole picture, and you can come back to the parts you feel you want to engage with some more. This book is packed with practical strategies and resources that are linked throughout the text, and where you are on your journey will guide which resources, knowledge, movement or practices resonate most for you at any time.

Something to note. If, when reading, anything feels stressful to you or you don't feel ready to engage with a particular part, feel free to skip that section and come back to it when you're ready. As you'll see throughout the book, the main aim is to help you cool things down, not ramp things up. You'll notice me say more than once that we don't treat pain with more pain.

That being said, if you come to the book with an open mind and willingness to better understand your body, you'll make the most of the info in this guide.

You may come across new terms that you're not yet familiar with, so to make it as easy and accessible as possible to learn about your body, I've included a simple glossary at the back of this book for quick reference.

Who is this book for?

I understand that we all have many identities that shape our experiences, how we engage with the world and how the world engages back, especially as it relates to sexual orientation, gender identity, and gender expression. Throughout the book, the language, metaphors and examples I use are often geared toward cisgender males and have a masculine tone. However, I'd like to highlight before we begin that this book is written for *anyone with a penis who is experiencing pain*. While I do specify the anatomy, and sometimes the identification of our parts might be at odds with the identification of ourselves, this information is still helpful.

Okay, no more beating around the bush. Let's get to it and understand what persistent pelvic pain is all about and what you can do about it.

CHAPTER 1

WHAT PELVIC PAIN IS... AND WHAT IT'S NOT

In the medical world, you've probably most often seen pelvic conditions labeled as 'chronic' pelvic pain syndrome (CPPS) or chronic prostatitis (CP). Both are used frequently and are highly applicable in medical practice, but these terms are not always inclusive when it comes to having pain 'down there.'

In this book, you'll never see me address your pain as a 'chronic' condition. Why? Well, because when I hear the word 'chronic,' I think 'permanent' and that's not what your symptoms are. Changing the way you relate to your pain is the first step to recovery. Knowing that your symptoms are persistent but can be resolved is oh-so liberating. Those fears about maybe living with pain for the rest of your life can be put to rest. So, let's take the word 'chronic' out of your vocabulary starting right now.

WHAT IS PERSISTENT PELVIC PAIN?

Male pelvic pain sits in a lot of categories and comes with a lot of tags. Sorta like a smorgasbord list of symptoms that – medically speaking – classify whether you have persistent pelvic pain or not. Generally, the definition of 'chronic' pelvic pain syndrome is having perceived pain in structures related to the abdomen or pelvis lasting more than three to six months without a known cause or pathology that typically results in sexual health issues, urinary complaints and lots of worry to say the least.[3] [4] (I mean, it's your private parts we're talkin' about. Of course

1

it's worrying when you don't know what's wrong.) It's commonly a diagnosis of exclusion, meaning that through the process of elimination
(via lots of tests, procedures, and doctors visits), if there is no medically identifiable cause, CPPS/CP is the discerned diagnosis. 'Prostatitis'-
like issues are the most common urological cases seen in men less than
50-years-old.[5] [6] For the sake of consistency in what you read on the
internet and in books, male pelvic pain has been classified by the gov-
ernment research organization National Institute of Health (NIH) as
'chronic prostatitis.' This is a bit of a misnomer, because in a majority
of cases the prostate isn't to blame – just an innocent bystander. In fact,
greater than 90% of 'prostatitis'-like symptoms fall under the umbrella
of chronic pelvic pain syndrome.[7] [8]

If you want to get real technical, the NIH classifies 'prostatitis' into
four categories:[9]
1. Acute bacterial prostatitis
2. Chronic bacterial prostatitis
3. Chronic non-bacterial prostatitis
    a. inflammatory
    b. non-inflammatory
4. Asymptomatic inflammatory prostatitis

For decades, 'prostatitis' has been a clinical enigma for healthcare providers, and to this day we lack a universal definition and language to
describe it. To put your mind at ease, any word with '-itis' at the end of
it technically means inflammation, but this doesn't necessarily mean
that inflammation or an infection is the cause of your pain. Don't get
me wrong. The immune system does play an important role in your
pain experience, but it's just one of many protective mechanisms involved. More on this later.

Now, 90-95% of persistent pelvic pain cases are classified as Type
III chronic non-bacterial prostatitis or CPPS.[10] [11] The most important
take-away message is that approximately 5%-10% of cases might be
caused by an active bacterial infection, which means the likelihood of
a bacterial infection causing the problem is questionable.[12] Typically
(but not always), when there's an infection present, you might have

symptoms of fever, chills, general ache, malaise, genital pain, pain with urination, sudden changes in urinary urge, blood in urine, and there may be evidence of opportunistic (infectious and potentially harmful) bacteria in prostatic secretions or urine when viewed under a microscope. White blood cell (WBC) count can be elevated with an acute infection, but it can also be elevated in inflammatory non-bacterial prostatitis, for which the treatment approach remains the same as CPPS.[13] Interestingly, men who don't have symptoms of CPPS/CP can also have increased white blood cell count and positive opportunistic bacteria cultures show up on diagnostic tests.[14]

When bacterial '-itis' is highly suspected, antibiotics like fluoroquinolones, the most commonly prescribed, have shown to be an acceptable treatment option for acute or chronic bacterial prostatitis and should clear things up 40-90% of the time.[15][16] The wide range of elimination rates reported varies based on the type of antibiotic (or combination) used in the study and the uniqueness of the individual taking the medication. Everyone has their own particular architecture. Unfortunately, there are many variables involved when it comes to determining the efficacy of any treatment, so we have to scrutinize statistics and make treatment recommendations on a case-by-case basis. This is why no one single treatment option works for every single body.

Although antibiotics have been widely accepted as a treatment option for bacterial prostatitis when it is highly suspected to be present, it should not require several rounds of antibiotics for treatment. In doing so, there is a risk of building resistance to antibiotics, meaning they become less effective when you really need them. Not to mention the reported side effects experienced by some who take them, this discrepancy having to do with genetic variability, according to some scientists' proposals. Consequences of frequent and prolonged antibiotic use reported in the literature include disruption of cellular health and protective microorganisms, systemic effects on the nervous and musculoskeletal systems, and altered organ function.[17] So, if you've already had an unsuccessful round of antibiotic treatment, suffice to say, it's better to use medication only when you actually need it. Currently, antibiotic therapy is recommended for initial consideration if you haven't been exposed to very much antibiotic treatment, have a history of urinary tract infections (UTIs), or had really good results with a short bout of antibiotic treatment in the past.[18]

If not treated appropriately, acute bacterial prostatitis could become persistent, which is a further reason to exercise caution around antibiotics. Frequent infections (pelvic related or not) due to an alerted immune system can also alter the sensitivity of nerves around pelvic organs and surrounding tissues. And when your alarm bells go ringing, pelvic muscle tension and pain might be just one of many protective responses you experience. The more these protective patterns happen, the harder it might be to 'let go' of tension down there or even be aware of it. These are normal responses to have. And the best part is, you can work on them.

All in all, the real question to ask is: Why are you getting these infections in the first place? What can be done to support your body's immune function? Stay curious, because there's more to come on supporting your immune system in the All Systems Go chapter.

IS IT AN INFECTION?

I'd recommend getting in touch with a healthcare provider specializing in urologic health, who takes the time to listen to your story and looks at your case with a wide-lens approach. It's wise to make sure there isn't anything more serious going on.

If you're in the clear on the big stuff, you could ask for a two-glass pre-massage and post-massage test before taking the antibiotics route. This involves taking samples of mid-stream urine and post-prostate-massage urine to indicate the presence of a 'true' bacterial infection. A post-prostate-massage urine sample is a pee sample after the doctor massages the prostate to include prostate specific fluids. Studies show this test is 96% effective in identifying potentially harmful bacteria in the prostate.[19] If there is a notable increase in WBCs present when samples are compared for opportunistic bacteria under a microscope, it could mean a bacterial infection.

However, it's also completely normal to have a few WBCs and opportunistic bacteria in prostatic fluid. As mentioned earlier, there are individuals who are symptom-free but their diagnostic tests show otherwise. Since we're on the topic of bacteria, it's worth noting that there have been reports of urethral microbiome differences observed with first void urine samples. Although these differences are present, it's still not clinically indicative of pathology, but perhaps this tells us that there might be a change in the overall bacterial ecosystem balance.[20] Biomarkers for CPPS/CP aren't so cut and dry. They are just one piece of a very complex puzzle and should be taken into account considering your individual concerns and symptom presentation. If the results come back positive, you and your health provider may decide it's a green light to treat with antibiotics appropriately tailored to address your individual case.

The point I'm making here is that diagnostic tests can be helpful if your health provider takes them into consideration with the whole picture. There are limitations with diagnostic tests as they are not 100% accurate 100% of the time. We are also limited by what technology and our understanding of these complex systems can currently provide and offer. There might even be factors we haven't discovered yet.

Many men have never had their prostate or semen fluids checked to rule out infection, but even if they were tested and results came back negative, they were still treated with multiple rounds of antibiotics anyway.[21] Here's why that's a problem. What happens is you'll feel good for a short period of time because all antibiotics have a pain-relieving effect, but then the symptoms return, sometimes even worse than before. In fact, one study noted that the more treatments and procedures someone has had for CPPS/CP, the worse their reported outcomes for pain and quality of life.[22] It's important that the provider you're seeing doesn't mask your symptoms by throwing a bunch of meds at you. This kind of treatment is like throwing spaghetti at a brick wall. Nothing sticks for long.

Bottom line: Antibiotics don't cure persistent pelvic pain.

WHAT IF IT'S NOT AN INFECTION?

If you don't have an active infection, like in up to 95% of cases, it's most likely Type III chronic non-bacterial prostatitis (with or without inflammation), otherwise known as chronic pelvic pain syndrome. Why the difference in these two names though? (After all, I promised never to use the word 'chronic,' didn't I?) Well, the NIH changed the name of this category from prostatitis to pelvic pain or CPPS, because the symptoms that you experience might not be coming from your prostate at all. And in my experience, this is often the case.

Don't let that word 'inflammation' fool you into thinking this isn't stress-related. Pain in the nether regions will trigger the stress response mechanisms that influence your immune function. Most often, the presence of inflammation doesn't have a direct correlation to the severity or number of symptoms you experience.

Although the symptoms themselves are distressing, it's the resultant suffering that really has an impact on men's lives. Like mood changes, worrisome thoughts, feelings of anxiety or frustration, altered libido and sexual enjoyment, difficulty concentrating at work, difficulty participating in life (which might look like reducing social and physical activities, relationship challenges, less ability to be involved with family, feeling like no one takes you seriously and not having a healthcare provider you can trust to guide you in the right direction). There are many men with pelvic pain who feel this way. In fact, 140 men from 39 different countries who participated in the development of a new assessment tool measuring the impact of pelvic pain share the same sentiment.[23] What you're experiencing is normal.

It's not just the residual effects of pelvic pain that shape your experience, either. Your beliefs and thoughts about pain, your previous experiences with pain, your expectations and learned behavior from watching caretakers, what you've heard, read or seen from others' response to pain, especially those dealing with a similar issue, social taboos, and even religious views about your private parts are all involved. For some men, embarrassment further discourages them from talking about it with family, friends, partners, employers, and sometimes even healthcare professionals.

There are complex pathways interconnected between the body, spinal cord, brain, and your mind. Information is constantly being relayed, adjusted, and analyzed by your brain on a moment-to-moment basis. Your brain weighs the world for you. How it does that will depend on the extent of actual and/or perceived 'threats' you might be experiencing. And your brain will make predictions about the amount of protection you need based on your previous experiences.

Pain is a conscious, inner world experience. Conscious and subconscious processes influence our perception of danger and safety, pleasant and unpleasant, and, importantly, our experience of pain. The relational meaning that pain has for us as a human being, as a person experiencing the world from our own side, will be unique to us. In other words, we experience the world uniquely. What feels amazing for one person might feel horrid for another. You can apply this to almost anything in your own life and notice for yourself.

All this to say, any of these pathways and processes (known and unknown) can turn up or turn down the sensitivity of the overall system and need for protection.[24]

So, how would your outlook change if pain was not the metric you used to measure success and recovery? Perceived social support, pain coping skills and overstressing thoughts better predict quality of life than pain scores do.[25]

WHAT DOES IT FEEL LIKE?

Given CPPS covers so many potential categories, what does it even feel like? Persistent pelvic pain can include a combination of any of the following:

- ➤ Groin pain
- ➤ Tailbone or butt pain
- ➤ Burning or sharp pain at the tip, shaft, or base of the penis
- ➤ Urethral pain
- ➤ Feeling like your penis is 'engorged', 'hard', 'rubbery', 'uncomfortable', 'veiny', 'alien', or 'weird'
- ➤ Pain during or after ejaculation
- ➤ Pain during or after urination
- ➤ Ache in the scrotum or rectum
- ➤ Tight and tense feeling in scrotum, penis or rectum

➤ Feeling of pressure in the prostate or rectum
➤ Pain while sitting
➤ Having to pee all the time
➤ Abdominal pain
➤ Testicle or scrotal discomfort
➤ Pain between scrotum and anus
➤ Lower back pain
➤ Pain during sex
➤ Finding it impossible to sleep through the night without waking up to pee
➤ Feeling like you don't empty your bladder all the way
➤ Changes in urine stream
➤ Discomfort with bowel movements
➤ Straining with bowel movements

If you're experiencing any of the symptoms listed above, keep reading.

When you're not feeling good down there, anxiety, fear, depression and despair can tend to settle in, especially if you've had these symptoms for years without a solution. It's enough to scare anyone shitless. Studies report that men with persistent pelvic pain have greater rates of depression and a poorer quality of life overall.[26] [27] [28] And I'm not surprised. When your genitals aren't working or feeling like you think they should, it can seem like the definition of your manhood is at stake. I mean, how often do you talk about your junk in the locker room? Probably never, right? Many just don't talk about these things, which makes them feel more isolated, vulnerable, and alone when dealing with pelvic pain. The result? Relationships with family, friends, and partners suffer and social isolation kicks in. One study reported that the partners of men with pelvic pain had greater rates of pain during sex too.[29] Let's dissect this a bit more, shall we?

Like other species, humans are copycats by nature. Preliminary research by a group of Italian scientists discovered special neurons within the brain called 'mirror neurons' that activate when you do an activity, watch someone else doing the activity or even just think about the activity.[30] Take a yawn, for example. When you notice the person next to you yawn, why do you feel like yawning too? Or when you see someone else looking at their cell phone, you might have the urge to do the same. That's because your brain is mimicking their activity as if you were the one taking part in the activity. The ability for your brain to do the activities you love (and also those you find unbearable) requires thousands of brain networks in synchrony to make it happen, sorta like a laser beam light show.

The same goes for mirroring someone else's emotions. When someone starts laughing so hard they have tears running down their face, you start laughing just as hard (and hopefully, not peeing in your pants). When someone smiles at you, you've got the urge to smile back. Emotions can be contagious and so can pain. There's even been reports of fathers-to-be experiencing pregnancy symptoms, like morning sickness, weight gain, indigestion, rashes, constipation and even enduring labor pains. This phenomenon has its very own 'syndrome' named after it called Couvade syndrome.[31] All this to say, "If seeing someone in pain or talking about their pain activates our own mirror systems, remember to make sure that when you are with others in pain, you don't spend all your time talking about your pains."[32] Don't get me wrong, sometimes a brooding party is necessary, but don't stay long after the party has already ended. Use social support to lift your spirits, fill up your hope tank when things get rough, and find yourself a sounding board for effective strategies to help you use your mirror neurons to your advantage.

SO, IT ISN'T A SEX THING?

When you're in pain, the last thing you want to think about is sex. So, it's no wonder sexual trouble is part of the pelvic pain package that you didn't sign up for. Your penis doesn't have a mind of its own and won't just get an erection upon command. Sorry to burst your bubble!

Let's say, for example, you're a 26-year-old with burning pain at the tip of your penis, and every time you ejaculate, you get this terrible gnawing ache in your crotch. You don't have any pain getting an erection or during intercourse, but you have more and more trouble 'getting it up' and now you're freaking out. You get increasingly frustrated and are worried that you're not 'normal.'

What really went on when you were trying to get it on? Were you scared about performing? Anxious that you'll be in agony for the next couple of days after sex? How's your self-esteem? Worried that your partner's going to find out something's 'wrong' with you? As I mentioned before, these are legitimate thoughts that many people have when they are experiencing this.

The NIH surveyed 488 men with CPPS/CP and found that 74% had ejaculatory pain at some point during their three-month study.[33] It's common to experience sexual difficulties while having pelvic pain. Unfortunately, sexual health issues can wreak havoc on your confidence, sexual identity, relationship with yourself and your partner, even causing anxiety that impacts other aspects of your life. We'll talk more about thoughts, pain and the brain in a later chapter, but for now here are a few common sexual concerns that you could be experiencing along with persistent pelvic pain:

- ➤ Low libido
- ➤ Trouble keeping an erection
- ➤ Difficulty with orgasm
- ➤ Low volume ejaculate
- ➤ Early or delayed ejaculation
- ➤ Pain with or after ejaculation
- ➤ Performance worry
- ➤ Changes in how your penis feels or looks when it's in a soft or erect state

WHERE THE HELL DID THIS PAIN COME FROM?

It's been said that up to one in every 6.25 men will experience symptoms of 'prostatitis' or pelvic pain at some point in their lives.[34] [35] There are lots of theories going around about persistent pelvic pain, none of which has been entirely proven. Most are just speculation based on anecdotal evidence or common features seen in research or clinical experiences. Just to be clear, there is no one known single cause for persistent pelvic pain. However, there are some triggers that might correlate with pain. The following list of potential triggers are not all-inclusive. It's also worth noting that there are people who experience some of these triggers and don't have persistent pelvic pain.

Potential triggers of pelvic pain:[36][37][38]

- ➤ Abdominal, pelvic, or genital surgery
- ➤ Sexually transmitted disease (STD) or infection
- ➤ Unrelenting stress
- ➤ History of unwanted sexual experience(s)
- ➤ Direct trauma to the pelvis or genitals (accidents, sports, crazy sexcapades)
- ➤ Infection of bladder, urethra, prostate and/or elsewhere
- ➤ Immune mediated or allergic response
- ➤ 'Cranky' pelvic tissues due to movement habits or mechanical tissue stressors
- ➤ Digestive issues like chronic constipation, irritable bowel syndrome (IBS), irritable bowel disease (IBD)
- ➤ Altered microbiota (living microorganisms) in intestinal and genitourinary tract
- ➤ A combination of any of the above

No matter what crazy stuff you've read on the internet, you didn't get pelvic pain from watching porn, masturbating, or 'bad' posture. It's worth knowing as well, in most cases, men with pelvic pain don't have an STD. The internet acts like a double-edged sword. It can be an outlet for social support and comradery with other people going through similar struggles, and in some cases can lead you to resources that are very helpful. That being said, exercise caution with what you read on the internet because it can serve to make you paranoid. I suggest putting your worries aside; they're only making matters worse.

Okay, enough of the background on pelvic pain and its discontents. It's time to get to know your privates.

CHAPTER 2

THE LOWDOWN DOWN BELOW

Urethra.
Coccyx.
Fascia.
What?!

Bet you're glad you signed up for this lesson! In order to better navigate your way through pelvic pain, you're going to need an understanding of how your bits and pieces work. The more you know about how your body works, the more confident you'll be in taking matters into your own hands, as it were. Let's get to it.

Pelvic floor function relies on the dynamic and interconnected relationship between bones, muscles, ligaments, organs, fascia, nerves and blood vessels.[39] Not to mention the synergistic coordination and function that it has with the rest of your body. Nothing lives in a vacuum, which is why this anatomy lesson starts with noticing these muscles on yourself.

You might feel things better if you do this sitting up nice and tall. Take your palm and put it underneath the area between your testicles and your anus. (You might also know this area as the taint – 't'ain't your balls and t'ain't your anus'.) You can reach from the front, back, or side, whatever feels most comfortable for you. Now, cough, or better yet, fake a loud laugh. (The laughter option will make you feel better! It's a great painkiller.)[40] What did you feel? You might've noticed some movement in your hand. Maybe a lift? Maybe a bulge? Regardless of what you felt, you just experienced first-hand the workings of your pelvic muscles. These muscles keep you from pooping in your pants during those deep kettlebell squats you might do at the gym. These (among other structures) make up your pelvic floor.

PELVIC FLOOR 101

Now we've located these crucial muscles, I'm going to take you through a quick anatomy lesson focusing on the importance of your pelvic floor, because there's more to your genitals than a cock and balls. In simple terms, you can think of the pelvis like a large cereal bowl, with the pelvic floor muscles making up the bottom of the bowl, extending from your pubic bone to your tailbone.

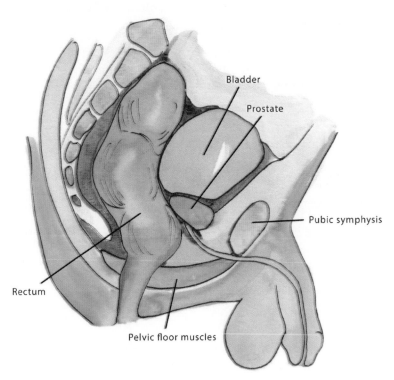

Side view of pelvic structures *in situ*

The pelvic floor plays a highly important role in your everyday physiological functions, like pooping, peeing, and sex. Let's summarize their job with what I call the Five 'S'es.

SPHINCTERIC CONTROL: The pelvic floor muscles clamp down on the tubes that empty your bladder and bowel to keep you continent. They relax when you pee or poop.

SUPPORT: These muscles support your abdominal and pelvic organs and work with your breathing muscle to regulate your body's intra-cavitary pressure systems. For example, when you cough, laugh, or sneeze, the pelvic muscles reflexively engage to work with the change in pressure coming down from your abdomen into your pelvis.

STABILITY: Pelvic floor muscles work together with the rest of your body to optimize movement and help with postural support and adaptability. The same as other skeletal muscles in your body, they're constantly adjusting and adapting to your activity and posture. Normally, you don't have to think about activating these muscles because a lot of these functions happen automatically, thank goodness!

SEXUAL APPRECIATION: Yes, you read that right. Your pelvic floor (the muscles as well as peripheral nerves, ligaments, blood vessels, spinal cord, and brain) helps with your ability to get an erection, keep an erection, and ejaculate. What about orgasms, you might ask? The most important organ involved with orgasm is the one sitting between your ears. Although often occurring at the same time, an orgasm is not ejaculation. It's a conscious and very visceral experience of your peak pleasure in that moment. There's no 'standard' feeling when it comes to orgasm. Everyone experiences orgasm differently, and each orgasm itself is unique.

SUMP PUMP: Just like any plumbing, you've got to have good flow down there. When you ejaculate, the pelvic muscles squeeze and release to pump out ejaculate fluid. "No matter how you shake or dance, the last few drops go down your pants." These muscles also help squeeze the penile urethra after peeing to get the last drops of urine out so you don't have to be embarrassed about dribbling pee on your pants.

There are three layers of muscle groups that make up the pelvic floor. We're going to start from the outermost layer and dive deeper to the innermost layer. Don't worry about pronouncing or memorizing all the names. All you need to know is that these tiny muscles exist and why they're important.

OUTERMOST LAYER

- ➤ Bulbospongiosus
- ➤ Ischiocavernosus
- ➤ Superficial transverse perineal
- ➤ External anal sphincter

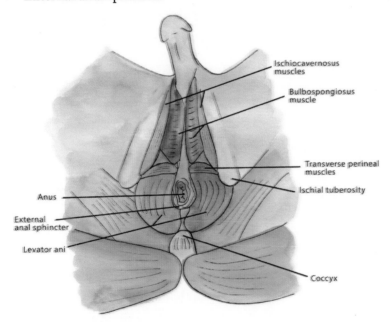

Outermost layer pelvic muscles

This group of muscles helps with orgasm, ejaculation, urination function (allowing the urethra and bladder to empty) and bowel function. Imagine those times when you need to fart, but you're in an elevator full of people; the external anal sphincter helps keep that fart in until you're safe to let loose.

Contrary to what you might think, the penis is actually soft erectile tissue made of three chambers. These chambers are porous, sort of like a sponge. It's designed this way so blood can fill the penis during erection and easily drain after ejaculation. Erectile tissues have attachments to the bony parts of your pelvis and share connections with the outer and middle layers of the pelvic floor muscles. When the penis fills with blood, the bulbospongiosus and ischiocavernosus muscles (located at the base of the penis) squeeze the chambers to help increase pressure within the erectile tissue, which helps keep the penis pumped with blood, giving you that 'hard-on' you know well.

You should also be aware that sexual function is a neurophysiological process that involves a collection of complex muscular, vascular, neural and molecular reactions to make a hard-on happen. Your brain, thoughts, and beliefs are also major players in the game.

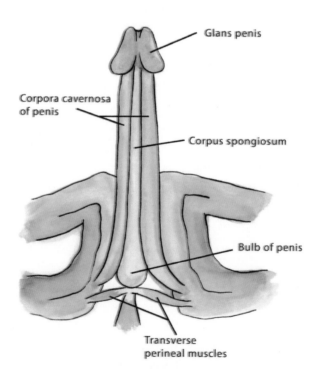

Erectile structures of penis

MIDDLE LAYER

➤ Deep transverse perineal
➤ Sphincter urethrae
➤ Compressor urethrae
➤ Perineal membrane (fibrous connective tissue that divides the middle layer from the outermost layer)

This group adds further support around the urethra to keep you from peeing yourself during times of exertion, strengthens fascial connections with your urogenital structures, and helps stabilize the pelvis and lower spine during movement.[41] There are also important neurovascular structures that run through the outer and middle layers. More on those later in this section.

DEEPEST AND INNERMOST LAYER

➤ Pubococcygeus
➤ Puborectalis
➤ Iliococcygeus
➤ Coccygeus

The diagram on page 18 shows the innermost layer of the pelvic floor, as viewed from the top. Imagine if I sliced you in half at your waist line and took the top off. What you'd see is the bottom of that cereal bowl I mentioned earlier.

Together, this group of muscles is called the levator ani, which literally means to 'lift the anus', and is also known as the pelvic diaphragm. These muscles support the pelvic organs (bladder, prostate, and rectum) that are also nestled in the pelvic bowl, and help you poop. These tiny little muscles are marathon runners. Their endurance and function are necessary to help reinforce the structural integrity of the pelvis provided by ligaments and connective tissue so things on the inside don't get saggy, so to speak.

Last but not least are the muscles that raise and lower your scrotum,

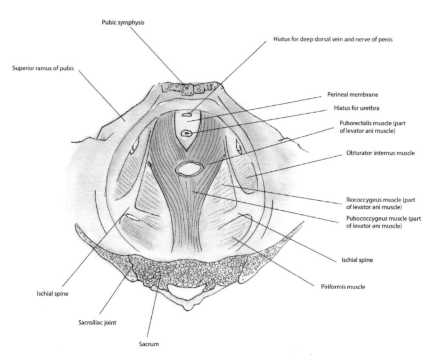

Pubic symphysis

Hiatus for deep dorsal vein and nerve of penis

Superior ramus of pubis

Perineal membrane

Hiatus for urethra

Puborectalis muscle (part of levator ani muscle)

Obturator internus muscle

Iliococcygeus muscle (part of levator ani muscle)

Pubococcygeus muscle (part of levator ani muscle)

Ischial spine

Piriformis muscle

Ischial spine

Sacroiliac joint

Sacrum

Innermost pelvic muscle layer

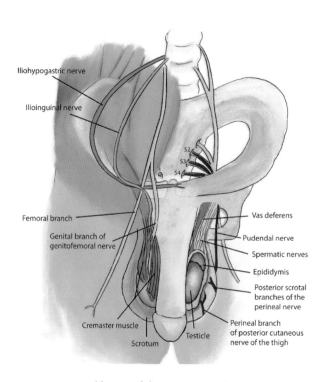

Iliohypogastric nerve

Ilioinguinal nerve

S2

S3

S4

Femoral branch

Genital branch of genitofemoral nerve

Cremaster muscle

Scrotum

Testicle

Vas deferens

Pudendal nerve

Spermatic nerves

Epididymis

Posterior scrotal branches of the perineal nerve

Perineal branch of posterior cutaneous nerve of the thigh

Nerves of the scrotum and testicles

which you can see in the diagram on page 18. The cremaster muscles (you've got one on each side of your sack) come from your internal oblique muscle (abdominal muscle), wrap around your spermatic cord and cradle each testicle. When you jump into cold water, you might experience some 'shrinkage.' These are your cremaster muscles hard at work protecting your little swimmers and ensuring optimal temperature for survival.

Also, you might notice that your scrotum raises or might get a little tense when you're aroused, about to ejaculate, or nervous. These are normal physiological responses that don't necessarily scream for your attention. Until they do...

IT'S NOT JUST ABOUT THE MUSCLES

Muscles are important, but in order for them to work together, there needs to be a communication highway that allows for effective function and coordination. Your nervous system has a lot to do with how your pelvic floor muscles work. The brain and neurons make up about 2% of the whole body but utilize 25% of the fuel (O2) and do most of the grunt work.[42] The nerves that supply your pelvic muscles mainly originate from sacral spinal nerves S2-S4. In fact, as you can see from the image on page 20, there are a lot of nerves in the pelvic region.

The job of the nerves is to relay messages from your tissues to your spinal cord, which then sends the messages on to your brain to interpret. This is important to know because nerves travel along bones, through connective tissue and muscles, and even within their own fascial tunnels. There are also nerves that supply nerves themselves! They move and stretch with you, and are pretty darn resilient. To say it frankly, the pelvis can tolerate a lot of pounding. (Just watch a video of a bull-riding competition if you don't believe me!) It has been said that the nerves of the pelvic floor can be stretched 6-22% of their original length before damage occurs![43]

That being said, sometimes nerves can become cranky. Blood vessels supply nourishment to nerves, and when these nerves aren't being fed or drained properly, they can get a bit ornery. Your tissues crave movement for nourishment so this is one way to help with 'cranky nerve syndrome.'

Before we get into what causes issues in your tissues, let's take a look at a few of the specific nerves that come into play. The pudendal nerve, the most commonly talked about with pelvic pain, is just one of many neural network highways that communicate with your privates. This nerve and its many branches contain motor, sensory and autonomic fibers (autonomic meaning that some of these nerve fibers communicate directly with your pelvic organs and function automatically, so that you don't have to worry about all the physiological underpinnings that happen under the hood). This is why it isn't uncommon to experience urinary issues, like urgency or bowel changes, or sexual issues tagging along with pelvic pain. The dorsal nerve to the penis (a branch of the pudendal nerve) assists in activating muscles involved with an erection, sensation to the erectile tissue and the skin over the shaft of the penis and the glans penis.[44] There are also contributions from the perineal branch of the pudendal nerve to the shaft of the penis, too.[45]

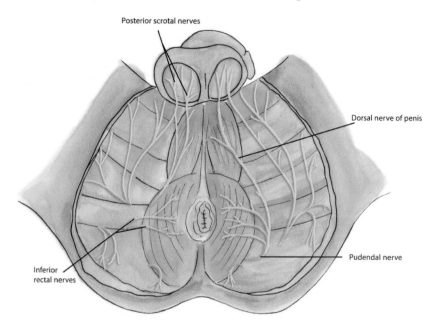

Nerves of male perineum

This is just a glimpse of the neuroanatomy of the pelvis. It does get a whole heap more complicated! What I'm driving at by talking about nerves, though, is that pain is a collective process, not a single source to reckon with.

When we map out the sensory nerves that supply the pelvic region, as in the picture on page 22, you can see the complexity and overlap that these nerve territories inhabit. These peripheral nerves emerge from your lower back and pelvic region to supply the skin and various structures of your pelvis, genitals, thighs, and butt. The nerves that supply these areas look after you and will report any suspicious behavior up to your spinal cord and then to the boss: your brain. Sometimes a nerve (or most likely, a group of nerves) can have a hissy fit and become sensitive, reporting the slightest changes in your tissue as *danger*. A nerve can be sensitive even without any injury to the nerve itself or the surrounding tissues and vice versa. There are also reports of individuals who have spinal cord abnormalities, and their nerve injuries show up on diagnostic tests but they don't experience pain.[46][47][48]

Pain is weird and complex. If a nerve does get cranky, it might feel tender to touch the area, and you might describe the feeling as burning, stabbing, or sharp. You might also feel a sudden 'zing' or a 'zap' without rhyme or reason.[49]

Nerve cells (also called neurons) throughout the body and those in your brain can also act like nosey neighbors. When your house alarm goes off, you might expect the police and fire department to arrive shortly after to check out the scene and make sure you're safe. The longer the commotion at your house goes on, the more curious your neighbors will get. Soon enough, they'll be out on your front lawn wondering what's happening, gossiping with the rest of the neighborhood. Nerves behave in a similar way. They adapt and recruit other nerve cells in neighboring areas to protect you, which may mean making things more sensitive so that they really grab your brain's attention. Great defense mechanism in the short term... not so great in the long term, especially when it relates to your most prized parts.

It's difficult, though tempting, to point the finger at just one nerve or just one single cause of pain. Truth is there's normal anatomical

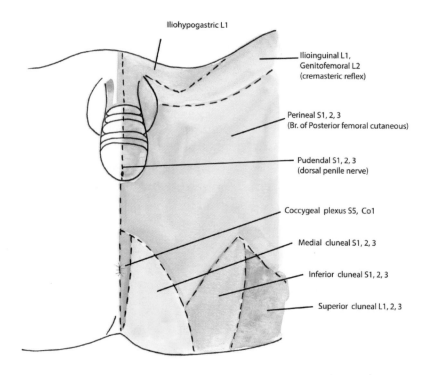

Iliohypogastric L1

Ilioinguinal L1,
Genitofemoral L2
(cremasteric reflex)

Perineal S1, 2, 3
(Br. of Posterior femoral cutaneous)

Pudendal S1, 2, 3
(dorsal penile nerve)

Coccygeal plexus S5, Co1

Medial cluneal S1, 2, 3

Inferior cluneal S1, 2, 3

Superior cluneal L1, 2, 3

(Adapted from Diane Jacobs): sensory nerves of male perineum

variations and interconnections between these nerves and other bodily structures. Just because we have naturally occurring anomalies and variations – much the same as trees – that doesn't mean that it's pathology or cause of pain.

In addition to the nerves I've mentioned, your testicles and scrotum are supplied by nerves coming from your lower back and sacrum (end part of your spine). In the image on the next page, you can see branching of nerves coming out from the lower back (lumbar nerves 1-5), running through multiple layers of abdominal connective tissue and muscles, and making their way to the skin at the front of the abdomen just above your pubic bone. Then there are those nerves I just spoke about that come from your lower back into the genital region, and all the way down to your scrotum and testicles as well.

Despite pain being incredibly complex, there is some good news in all this: you're not going crazy if you feel pain that travels all over the

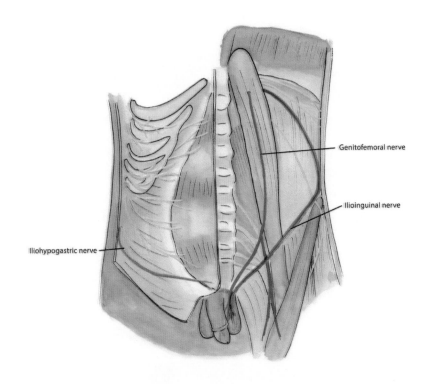

Nerves of the abdominal wall

place from your abdomen even down to your feet, because that highway extends all the way down there, too. Best yet, all of this is adaptable, workable and changeable.

But it's not just nerves in this mix when it comes to this communication. You've also got immune cells (and nerves cells that act like immune cells) patrolling all over your body making sure you're safe. These cells (including those in your brain) also have a sharp memory and will recognize anything that resembles a previous 'threat' or 'danger' associated with any context in your life (biological, psychological and or sociological) if deemed important enough to remember.[50] No two independent events are exactly the same, and these cells might activate to doubly protect you, just in case. Although the circumstances of life events might differ, these overly protective policemen might not pick up on that difference.

To put this in context, let's say you just got done with some

23

hanky-panky, then out of nowhere, you feel a not-so-familiar sensation in your penis. Of course, this is rather alarming because it's uncomfortable, foreign, and might even be associated with an incessant need to urinate (or some other weird bodily symptoms). The more these symptoms persist, the greater these areas grab your attention. Unknown to you, important neuroimmune mechanisms are already underway (taking record of this event for the future) to protect you. You might notice a change in your breathing, heart rate, muscle tension, maybe even changes in the way your penis looks and behaves. These changes are normal considering the circumstances, but an activity that was pleasurable has now become an activity of heightened concern. *Bam!* Just like that, learned associations are made. The more these associations play out (get reiterated), the more your protective systems will anticipate a negative outcome and do their best to predict future painful events.[51] As a result, you might find yourself caught up in worrying thoughts, changing your posture or movement patterns, and even avoiding activities you use to love.

The once-unconscious happenings in your underpants are now very much conscious; a physical and emotional response is now associated with this event, so anything that resembles this event can elicit similar psychophysiological responses. Persistent pain begins to shift from just a purely sensory experience into an emotionally driven process. Memories related to this experience and those that continue to reinforce this memory dig deeper grooves and patterns in the nervous system, which might be one of the many reasons why pain sticks around long after tissues have healed.[52]

Problematic molecular patterns can establish based on the type of bacteria, virus or illness involved, if any is present. Damage-associated molecular patterns can also occur.[53] This is where any damage to tissues elicits the release of certain chemicals involved in the healing process, which will be remembered by specialized immune and nerve cells. These can then activate in similar ways should circumstances resemble the prior experience of 'threat' again. Although these immune cells are necessary to protect you, unfortunately, they can be rather unselective. Go figure!

You even have maps in your brain (involved in motor and sensory processing) that are devoted to your body parts.[54] Scientists have coined this depiction of the body map the *homunculus*, which means 'little man' in Latin. Although the image below shows us as having clear-cut distinctions and 'real estate' mapped for certain body parts, in reality, it's not that simple. Generally, the larger the actual body part, the more brain cells are devoted to it, which means it 'owns' more real estate on our body map. Since they were discovered, we now realize there is a lot of overlap with these maps, too, that they communicate with multiple areas in the brain, and that the size of an area represented by your body part will own more real estate based on how often you use that body part, the intricacy of that function and even the importance and meaning of that body part in your life.[55]

The more fascinating fact is that these brain maps and connections change on a moment-to-moment basis. The more your brain practices something – like learning to ride a bike – the better and stronger these

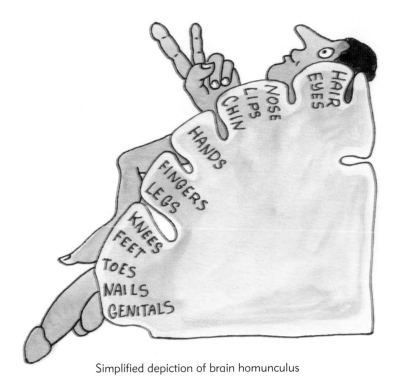

Simplified depiction of brain homunculus

25

connections get until it becomes automatic. The same process happens with pain. The more pain is 'practiced', the better your protective systems get at protecting you, even though you might not necessarily need it. Living with persistent pain can sometimes make you feel like your privates are foreign, different, and just downright weird. This might change the way that part of your body functions and how you relate to it. (For example, when things hurt down there, sex is not necessarily on your mind, so you might not be in the mood to play.) Although these altered sensations and body perceptions are scary to experience, rest assured that they're common with ongoing pain. Your brain and spinal cord change with pain, because the cells adapt to protect you, which sometimes means asking neighboring cells to help out (like running over to your neighbor's house and waking them up in the middle of the night).

When this happens, some confusion arises, and the body maps in your brain become less clear. It's like someone spilling coffee all over your trail map: you can hardly pick out the trail lines, but you still gotta move and head somewhere to get back to your car before the sun goes down. What started off as an easy hike is now a shot in the dark. Scientists call this loss of precision 'smudging'.[56] The less you use a body part, the more other neighboring brain cells get involved, and the less precise that part in the virtual body map in your brain gets, which can alter how that *actual* body part feels and functions. This might explain the weirdness that you can feel with your penis or the way the pain spreads and moves around as if it had a mind of its own.

As complicated as all this sciencey stuff may sound, know that your brain is constantly changing, and with some clever training, you can change your perception of pain. To learn more about brain 'smudging', check out this video: https://youtu.be/3QVAY5stO3U

Brain fried yet? Hang in there because we've got just a few more concepts to cover. Next up, the bladder.

The bladder is a stretchy balloon that sits right behind your pubic bone. Its neighbors are the rectum, prostate, pelvic floor muscles, penis, and intestines. In fact, pretty much everything in the surrounding area can influence the urinary subdivision.

So, let's say one of your neighbors' alarms goes off in the middle of

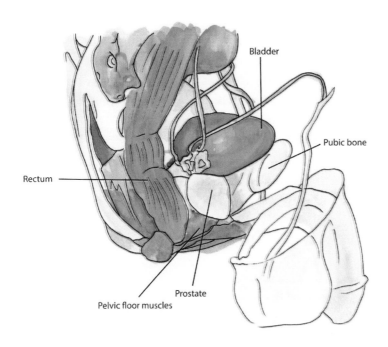

Male pelvic organs and neighboring structures

the night and keeps blaring until it wakes you up. Most likely, you'd flip on the lights and go see what the heck is going on next door, right? The same goes for the communication between the pelvic floor and your pelvic organs. Neighbors can be nosey, so when one house on the block is causing commotion, the others get curious, start peeking through the curtains and getting involved.

It's been said that there are over 45 miles of nerves in our body, communicating with our internal and external world.[57] Whenever there is distress, you better believe these nerves are going to perk up and listen. Pelvic pain is distressing, and this causes the alarm bells to keep going off, which can make neighboring structures curious indeed, sometimes even joining in the commotion.

You may or may not experience urinary symptoms – such as urgency, frequency, painful peeing – along with pelvic pain. If you don't, you're one of the fortunate ones. But if you do, don't sweat it because urinary issues are a common complaint associated with pelvic pain. Urgency and frequency (and pain) that isn't attributable to infection or known pathology is most likely due to an overly sensitive nervous system.[58]

Even in the cases of diagnoses like interstitial cystitis (IC) or bladder pain syndrome (BPS), we're discovering that the neuroimmune system plays an integral role. Many of the same symptoms overlap with those we see in pelvic pain, which is why diagnosis isn't so easy and misdiagnosis is common.

Pelvic pain symptoms overlapping with IC/BPS include:
- ➤ Pressure or discomfort in the lower belly
- ➤ Urinary urgency and frequency
- ➤ Painful urination
- ➤ Peeing making it feel better or worse
- ➤ Bladder spasms
- ➤ Bladder pain

These are umbrella symptoms that can fall under many categories and shouldn't be treated with a 'find it and fix it' approach. Urinary symptoms are multicausal and can often co-occur with pelvic pain. Things that can make the bladder unhappy might include constipation, non-relaxing pelvic floor muscles, and an upregulated nervous system, just to name a few. It's important to note that diagnoses like IC or BPS are still poorly understood. Rest assured, though: the initial course of action should be on the less invasive side. You can discuss this with your health professionals if this diagnosis applies to you.

If you haven't caught on yet, your bladder doesn't live in a vacuum. To help you feel better about your bladder woes, let's go over how your bladder actually works. The bladder is a storage tank that fills and empties. The entire peeing process (called micturition) involves sophisticated and complicated neurophysiological mechanisms to make this happen. Thank goodness you don't have to think about these processes for them to occur. For most of us, we don't notice our bladder filling or think twice about peeing – other than the friendly reminder we feel letting us know that it's really time to go.

Now, this might be a different story when you have pelvic pain. Your attention is always on your privates. You become super attuned to the subtle sensations in your pants including the messages coming from your bladder.

Normally, as your bladder fills, the bladder muscle (detrusor) relaxes and your pelvic muscles responsible for sphincteric control keep the urinary tube closed so there are no accidents. *Phew!* At around 150-200ml full, your bladder begins to stretch, at which point you might be cognizant of the initial urge to pee. As your bladder continues to fill and reaches about 400-600ml, you'll get another, possibly stronger urge to pee. Amazingly, your bladder can hold about two cups of urine! When it's time to go, your pelvic muscles relax, the flood gates open and

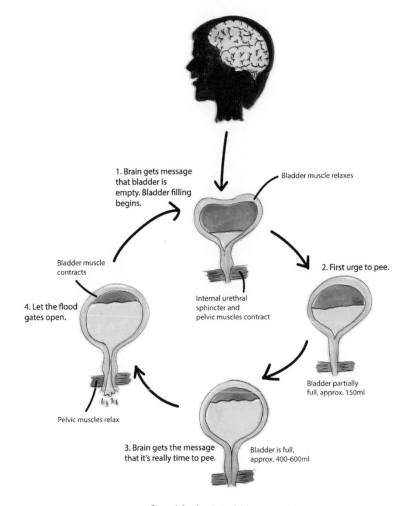

1. Brain gets message that bladder is empty. Bladder filling begins.

Bladder muscle relaxes

Bladder muscle contracts

2. First urge to pee.

4. Let the flood gates open.

Internal urethral sphincter and pelvic muscles contract

Bladder partially full, approx. 150ml

Pelvic muscles relax

3. Brain gets the message that it's really time to pee.

Bladder is full, approx. 400-600ml

Simplified micturition process

your bladder empties with some squeezing assistance from the detrusor muscle. At the end of this pee symphony, know that there's always going to be some residual urine left over in your bladder, up to 50ml.

The actual perceived sensation or urge to pee comes from your brain as it receives messages from your bladder and accompanying structures involved in the peeing process. As mentioned earlier, sometimes these messages can get confused, overly sensitive and extra obvious on your radar, which can heighten your stress and anxiety over your bodily functions. This sense of lack of control over your bodily functions is no doubt stress-inducing, but know that these issues are not permanent and can be trained back to your normal.

EVER HEARD OF KEGELS?

Checking in with your body is a good self-assessment practice. From the exercise you did at the beginning of this chapter, you know where your pelvic floor muscles are and what they do. The walk-through that we did was similar to Kegels, which if you haven't heard, are just as important to practice as letting go.

Let's go over the exercise again, so you get familiar with how things are – shall we say – *hanging*. Start by standing naked in front of a mirror. Don't be shy. This is the best feedback you can get. Next, lift your 'nuts to your guts,' meaning try to lift the base of your penis without using your hands. Alternatively, you can think of this as shortening the base of your penis and tightening around the anus like you're stopping the flow of urine or holding back a fart. Another way of putting it is to 'flick' your penis up and down. (And no, I don't mean spinning your penis around like a helicopter!)

Did you manage it? How did it feel? What did you notice?

When you contract your pelvic floor muscles, you might notice the penis moving up and in, the anus lifting and closing, and the testicles lifting slightly. When you let go, all parts should move back down to their original position in a smooth transition. There should be a visible range of motion with no other muscles helping out. If you're doing it correctly, no one should be able to tell you're doing them, except for you.

Common mistakes with pelvic floor exercises can include:
➤ Squeezing your butt cheeks
➤ Squeezing your thighs
➤ Tightening your abs
➤ Holding your breath
➤ Pushing down
➤ Giving 100% all the time. Too much of a good thing can lead to a habitual pattern of overactive or non-relaxing pelvic floor muscles which could make symptoms worse.

Notice how your pelvic floor muscles feel and function. If you're doing a pelvic floor contraction and your dangly bits aren't moving very far, you might have some weakness or non-relaxing pelvic floor muscles that don't let you contract any more; you may need to improve your overall awareness and motor coordination of these muscles. Perhaps you find yourself contracting your muscles correctly, but have a difficult time letting go or feel a jerking sensation. If so, this might be a sign of non-relaxing pelvic muscles too. Alternatively, you might find yourself doing the complete opposite, which means you're bearing or pushing down instead of contracting your pelvic floor muscles.

Being able to perform a pelvic muscle contraction correctly can be difficult if you lack awareness about your pelvic floor muscles, but being able to identify your pelvic floor is critical for everything else that's coming up. So, stick with it! I'm walking you through these steps in so much detail because being in tune with what you're feeling down there is an important way to self-assess and start making positive progress.

Do you remember the song *Dem Bones*? You know the one that goes: *The back bone connected to the thigh bone... The thigh bone connected to the knee bone... The knee bone connected to the leg bone...* Here's the (not so) subliminal message: it's all connected! The same goes for the pelvic floor muscles. In fact, your hips, spine, legs, abdominal muscles, diaphragm (breathing muscle), immune system, digestive system, vascular system, pelvic organs, peripheral nerves, spinal cord, brain, and more (just in case I forgot something) all have intimate connections with the pelvic floor. If you want to be successful at treating pelvic pain,

31

you've got to look at the big picture and not just focus on the bits that hurt.

THE DIAPHRAGM-PELVIC-FLOOR CONNECTION

The diaphragm is a dome-shaped muscle that sits underneath your rib-cage and is one of the primary muscles used for breathing. It has connections with your abdominal muscles, ribs, lower back and with vital

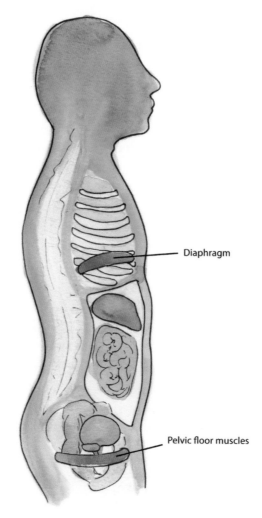

Diaphragm pelvic floor connection

organs like your liver, lungs and stomach. The diaphragm is involved in postural control and stability, in addition to respiratory control, fluid dynamics and regulating pressure systems in the body.

There's much more to breathing than just air moving in and out of your lungs for the body to take in oxygen. Breathing is a symphony of many neurophysiological interactions and is an activity that you can have some control over. Breathing assists with vascular and lymphatic flow and gives your abdominal organs a nice massage.[59] It has the ability to influence your physiological wellbeing and mental flexibility. In other words, you can use your breath to modulate higher brain centers involved in thinking, decision-making, emotions, and your sense of inner wellbeing and peace. The nerves that supply the diaphragm project to areas of the brain that are associated with emotions, autonomic function, and processing and integration of sensory and motor information.[60][61] Neural processes that help regulate the calming part of your nervous system also modulate your breathing patterns and vice versa. Several areas of the brain also feed forward information to your body in response to your environment, the sensory information perceived, and your internal state of being.

Since your breath can influence your nervous system (and vice versa), it can also influence your pain perception, emotions and experiences, as many of the same areas of the brain that respond to pain and emotions also share neural networks with breath control. Intentionally tapping into the sensations of your breath in a non-reactive and non-judgmental way provides an opportunity to build trust in your own sensory experiences, which turns down the sensitivity dial and turns up the safety dial. Neuroscientists who study pain investigated the effects of slow-paced breathing and mindfulness on pain intensity and found that intentional focus on breath sensations can reduce perceived pain intensity and unpleasantness via brain neural circuits independent of the body naturally producing endorphins (AKA painkillers).[62][63] This is important because your body's natural production of endorphins has been shown to modulate pain, and it's been postulated that breathing influences these neurochemical mechanisms. Of course, this is just one of the few studies available that demonstrate how purposeful attention to breath sensations influences pain perception and underlying physiological processes. Most likely pain relief is driven by both your naturally produced painkillers and changes in brain neural circuitry. Keep in mind that the exact neurophysiological mechanisms of breathing on pain and pain on breathing have yet to be fully understood.

You might have heard of diaphragmatic breathing, also known as deep belly breathing, used to ease pelvic pain. Realistically, we're always using our diaphragm to breathe so this is no different. The distinction might be whether or not we are intentionally aware of our breath or purposefully choosing to manipulate our breath to achieve some psychophysiological benefit.

There's also a synergistic interplay between breathing and pelvic muscle function: a natural movement of your pelvic muscles when you breathe.[64] When you breathe in, the pelvic floor muscles expand down and away; then when you breathe out, the pelvic floor muscles return to their natural resting position. We can use our breath to mobilize tissues of the pelvic diaphragm naturally and enhance bodily awareness, which in itself can create a sense of safety for our nervous system.

How much movement is normal? Well, nobody can objectively quantify this as yet. There is no normative measurement of relaxation or contraction of the pelvic floor muscles. As such, it's entirely based on your perception of what you feel in your own body. There will always be some inherent tone in your muscles. Having tension in your pelvic muscles isn't necessarily something that should alarm you. Activity of muscles is constantly changing and adapting in response to your internal and external environment in addition to whether or not you think the pain in your pants poses a threat. Naturally, when you are worried, frustrated or angry, your body will reflect these emotions, which may mean increased muscle tension that could be felt in your pelvic muscles and elsewhere in your body.

Pain demands attention whether or not actual tissue damage or injury is present. Shifting your attention towards and away from pain helps integrate higher cortical areas of the brain to decrease the influence of subcortical brain areas involved with emotional regulation and survival. One of the ways to do this is intentional focus on your breath, slooooww and steady.

A POSITION ON POSTURE

Here are two important messages about posture that I want you to know: perfect posture doesn't exist; and 'bad' posture doesn't equal pain. If you don't believe me, search 'strongmen lifting atlas stones' and check out their postures and variability in lifting the 353lb (160kg) stone. If lifting with a straight back is what you're 'supposed to' do to keep your back healthy and prevent pain, then how do you explain this? If there were a perfect way to do things that everyone should adopt, we would all be in trouble. That's not how we're built to function and live in the world. Your posture, movements, body mechanics and ability to adapt and change are entirely unique to you and your own individual architecture. So, let's take the words 'supposed to' out of your vocabulary.

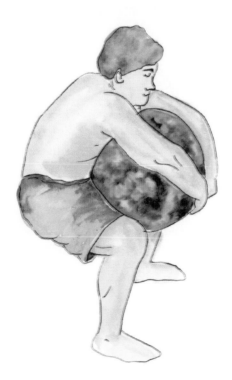

It's okay. Go ahead and pick up your jaw up off the floor. This should make you breathe a sigh of relief, because it means you don't have to worry about alignment or holding yourself in one rigid posture for fear that it'll make your pain worse. Your posture is constantly changing and adapting in your day based on what you see, what you do, what you think, who you're with, how you're feeling and so on. Don't get me wrong, posture might play a role in your symptoms, especially if you find yourself in positions that aggravate them or aren't moving much, AKA couch potato syndrome.

Let's try something. Go ahead and slouch. Now try taking a deep breath in. What does it feel like? Next, sit up tall and try taking a deep breath. What does that feel like? What did you notice between the two? Maybe you noticed that it's easier to take a deeper breath in while sitting up tall and relaxed than it is slouched and all scrunched up. That's because, in *some* cases, posture and how we move in the world *does* influence our physiology. Even your mood can be reflected with your posture. If you're scared, hurt or nervous, the chances of you sitting up tall with confidence are probably low. Just reflect on your own experiences around your posture and how your body moves in response to your mood, pain, and so on. What does your body feel like when you're happy or excited, when you're angry, sad or hurt? Pain is a motivator for change. It will impact the way you move, hold your body, breathe, and the actions you choose to take or not take. Some of these changes are conscious, but mostly they're subconscious. This is a normal, protective response.

While posture and its connection to emotion is interesting, numerous research studies suggest that posture isn't to blame for pain.[65][66][67][68] In fact, when you observe how 'healthy' people without pain sit, they're often found slouching![69] This also includes thinking that your pelvis is 'tilted,' or your pelvis is 'out of alignment,' or your core is 'weak,' and that any one of these is the cause for your troubles. Because it isn't. We all have our unique natural human variances and asymmetries. So, let's stop pathologizing what's normal.

When it comes to posture, variability in your day-to-day movements and positions does promote healthy nourishment for all your tissues including your brain, but no need to overwhelm yourself with unhealthy beliefs about posture. Instead, have fun with your posture, find ways to move that feel good to you, and most importantly don't worry whether you're doing it right or wrong. Remember, there's no perfect anything.

That was a lot of information in this section so it's okay if you didn't get a grip on all of it in one sitting. I encourage you to re-read this section as many times as you need to so that you feel comfortable understanding the complexities that underlie pain. Pain is weird, and it gets particularly complex when it has to do with your genitals. From an evolutionary standpoint, pooping, peeing and sex are vital physiological functions so it's no wonder that pain in your pelvis is nerve-wracking.

Okay, now that we're done with the nitty gritty nerve stuff, it's time to dive into the depths of your brain. Learning about how your brain works when in pain will be key for your recovery, because if you can get your brain on board, your body is bound to follow. You may think your penis has a mind of its own, but the next chapter is focused on that all-important organ. Your brain.

CHAPTER 3

GOT YOUR BODY ON THE BRAIN

You know that feeling you get when you whack your funny bone? I've done it a bunch of times. Does it send me cross-eyed? Sure. Do I know it's going to go away after I shake it off? Yup, no biggie. Why doesn't this pain last for weeks? Well, for one, I've whacked it before and know what to expect. Second, I can visibly see what's going on. Other people can relate, so the brain concludes this isn't a dangerous situation.

Here's the thing about pelvic pain that I really want you to know more than anything else in this book. Pain in the pelvis isn't permanent. Let me repeat that. Despite what people tell you, despite what you read on the internet, pain in the pelvis is not permanent. Pain anywhere in your body doesn't have to be permanent. We all experience pain. Aches and niggles are a normal part of life. This may come as a shock to you, but pain doesn't always mean there's tissue damage or harm.

Okay, deep breath. I'm gonna take it a step further. You can have a tissue injury and experience *no* pain. Now, I know what you're thinking. *Whoa, wait a second. You're telling me that pain doesn't come from my tissues? So, where does it come from? There's got to be something causing my pain.*

You probably think I'm crazy right now. And maybe I am a little, but not about this. Trust me (and the brave scientists and clinicians who've paved the understanding of pain science knowledge for decades now). If I'm crazy, how do you explain this? In 2014, the *Huffington Post* published an article 'Knife Falls From Sky Into Chinese Man's Head.' In it, a Chinese man was casually strolling the block, when out of no-where, a knife fell into his head. He said he felt 'a very heavy weight,' but

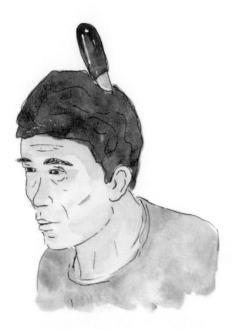

it wasn't until a bystander pointed out that a knife was stuck in his head that the pain went from feeling just 'heavy' to excruciating.

Or how about a war veteran who had shrapnel in his scrotum from a gunshot wound that he didn't know about for years until he went through a metal detector at the airport? True story! How do we explain pain in individuals who are born without a limb, but still experience pain in a limb that never existed to begin with?[70]

And then there's this one, my own personal experience. When I was 13 years old and playing basketball with my friends, my brother thought it would be fun to ride his bike right through the middle of our game. I noticed his bike had a sharp object sticking out of it, so I told him to go ride somewhere else, warning him that someone could get hurt. Well, that unlucky someone who got hurt was me! Except I had no clue when or how long my lower leg was sliced open! Only when someone told me I was bleeding did I look down at my leg and notice my calf muscle exposed. I fell to the ground in agony. Suddenly, it hurt like hell. It still baffles me that I didn't feel any pain until someone brought the injury to my attention!

Luckily, our Chinese friend turned out alright and my leg healed, but the point of telling you these stories here is to demonstrate that the sensations you feel change based on the context of any given situation. How your brain weighs the world for you in that moment will influence your perception of what's happening to you as a person and to your body. In my case, I was too busy having fun playing basketball with my friends, and it was more important for me to win the game and stay in the moment than to pay attention to the wound. It wasn't until someone spoiled the fun, letting me know that my lower leg was gushing blood, that my attention and focus changed because of the credible information provided to me; not only from what was happening in my tissues but also the context of my environment.

Take a moment now to think of a time in your life or in the life of someone you know who's had a similar experience with pain. If you're having a tough time thinking of something, just remember the last time you found a bruise on your body and had no idea where it came from; another perfect example of having tissue injury but experiencing no pain. Pain is weird!

Dr. David Butler and Prof. Lorimer Moseley, clinical pain scientists and educators, wrote a fantastic book called *Explain Pain*, which I highly recommend reading. Your pain levels might reduce just by reading this book. Interestingly, we have some research that supports when people in pain learn more about pain and increase their understanding about how it works, alongside relevant therapies, it can be more effective at relieving pain than current medications commonly used to treat persistent pain.[71] [72] [73] [74]

THE BRAIN ON PAIN

With persistent pain, the central nervous system (your brain and spinal cord) play an important role in filtering and processing sensory information from your external and internal environment. According to the International Association for the Study of Pain, pain is defined as 'an unpleasant sensory and emotional experience associated with, or resembling that associated with, actual or potential tissue damage.'[75] Pain is a normal human experience.

Pain is also an emergent process, not linear. That is to say: $X + Y \neq Z$. Can you find lust in your genitals? How about love in your heart? Pain arises from a collection of complex interactions (internal and external) and not just from any one single cause or event. The pain that you feel doesn't just come from your tissues; all experiences are processed from your perspective, your sense of 'self' including your memories and previous experiences with pain from which everything else is derived and taken into account.

Pain is a distributed process across multiple brain areas. There's no 'pain center.' It's definitely abstract to think about your brain contributing to pain. For one, you can't see it or see how it works. Then there's the topic of consciousness, which has many unanswered questions. New discoveries about our brains and bodies are constantly being made, but for now let's keep things simple and understand that pain is a personal and conscious experience influenced by neural, chemical and molecular processes that are interdependently related to biological, psychological and social aspects of you as a human being.[76] You can think of neurological patterns and associations in the brain like an airline map. There are many memory traces, patterns and associations made on a moment-to-moment basis.

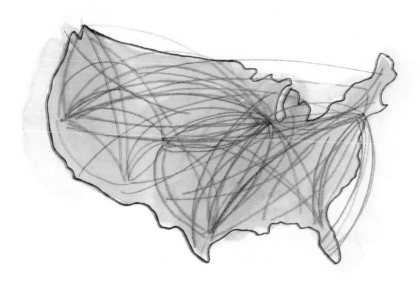

There's research to show that your brain actually changes with on-going pelvic pain. There's a unique neuronal activation pattern that is evident in those with chronic prostatitis/chronic pelvic pain syndrome.[77] This activation pattern was also shown to match up with pain intensity. One area in the brain that piques my interest with pain is called the insular cortex (insula). This is the integration hub that receives information from the external and internal environment. This part of our brain, in addition to others, integrates information from all other health systems of our body. The insular cortex is said to be the internal state detector of 'how am I feeling', checking in on your internal sense of wellbeing and self-awareness.

It's no surprise that the insula has connections with other parts of the brain involved in decision-making and emotional processing, including areas that mediate sexual motivation, fear, anxiety, reward, and pleasure.[78] Learning and long-term memory are also features of the insula; issues will get extra 'sticky' the more the event or recurring situation impacts your life or you as a person.[79] So, it's no wonder pain down under takes its toll! This gives us more proof of the suggestion that the central nervous system plays more of a role in the experience of pain and its persistence than what happens just at the tissue level.[80 81 82]

There are many different kinds of pain experiences and many different types of pain mechanisms involved in the narrative of pain, all of which are unique to you as an individual. The nitty gritty of this is too advanced to put into a book on pelvic pain such as this, but know that no two individuals experience pain in the same way, and there is no diagnostic test that can 'find' pain.

Don't get me wrong. Tissue issues can be a trigger that activates the alarm system, but not in isolation. Nothing lives in a vacuum. There are special sensory neurons called nociceptors that activate with harmful or potentially harmful chemical, mechanical, or thermal stimuli coming from your body and organs. Even if these sensory nerves activate, it doesn't mean that you'll experience pain. Depending on their location in the body, they behave and respond in different ways to different stimuli. Some sensors pass along messages at lightning speed and others at a slower pace. Think the tortoise and the hare. For example, if you stepped on a nail or had a knife fall out of the sky and stab you in the skull, you would want to know about it. It's a great protection system that is necessary for our survival.

These sensors send electrical impulses up to your spinal cord and then to your brain for further investigation. For example, when you're talking it up with your buddies, what's allowing you to hear what they're saying? You might've said your ear, and this is partially true. Your ear is a receptacle for sound to tunnel through, creating vibrations that stimulate little hair cells, exciting the nerves of your inner ear. This sends electrical signals to your brain to interpret those vibrations into words that you can actually understand. Fascinating, right?! Well, the same goes for the sensations that you feel in the body.

Those little sensors are found everywhere: in your skin, ligaments, joints, muscles, hair cells, bone, blood vessels, nerves, organs. The list goes on and on. These sensors respond to temperature, touch, pressure, stretch, movement, smell, sight, thoughts, stress and noise, and your brain is constantly sorting the important info from the unimportant. They're the same sensors that send messages up to your brain signaling actual or potential danger. Just like your brain makes sense of the sound that comes into your ear, it also perks up to potential 'danger' messages so that it can protect you. You'll experience pain if the brain decides it's important to have pain in that moment. Potential dangers can be *anything* that you perceive as a threat to your body or tissues, your lifestyle, sexuality, relationships, career, passions, or to you as a person. They can be physical like a venomous snake bite or they can be emotionally driven like the thought of your penis not working when you want to be sexually intimate. To learn more about the science of pain, check out this video: https://youtu.be/eakyDiXX6Uc

Any spot along this tissue-to-brain pathway can be involved in the perception of pain. Likewise, on several spots along this pathway, the 'danger' messages can be amplified and magnified. These neurological paths are interdependent and interconnected. Again, this proves how complex the pain process really is. It's really easy to blame it on pelvic muscles or the prostate, but when you really take a look at the literature, it's much more sophisticated than that.

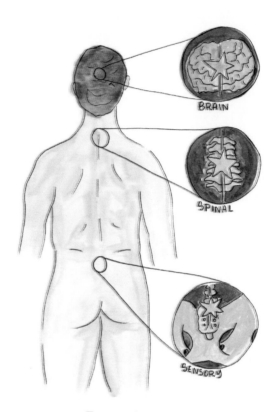

Tissue-to-brain pathway

Not all danger messages are harmful or the only cause for pain. In fact, you can have nociceptors activated and still not experience any pain.[83] Remember the amazing pain stories a few paragraphs back? If nociceptors keep activating alarm bells, this can perpetuate the flooding of 'danger' messages into the spinal cord and brain. There are many overlapping networks that fight for your attention and can keep these danger messages idling. Again, these are adaptive and protective processes that are vital for your wellbeing; process that are beneficial in the short term but not so helpful in the long term.

The perception of pain is influenced by a hodgepodge of factors, including but not limited to:

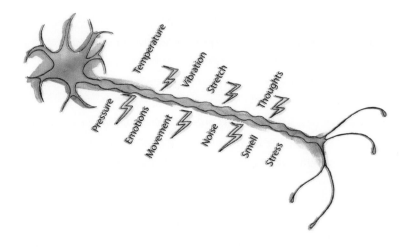

➤ Past experiences
➤ Learning
➤ Meaning of involved body part and the role it plays in your life
➤ Environment
➤ Beliefs
➤ Thoughts
➤ Values
➤ Fear
➤ Health status
➤ Tissue status
➤ Understanding and knowledge
➤ Safety
➤ Current context
➤ Expectations
➤ Perspective
➤ What you've been told
➤ Sociocultural taboos and stigmas
➤ Available support and resources
➤ Religion
➤ Spirituality

With persistent pain, the tissues have long since healed, but the message in your nervous system stays the same: that you're 'in danger.' When you have ongoing pain, the patterns and emotional memory traces get really good at playing the same tune to protect you.

As far back as 1949, neuropsychologist Donald Hebb postulated that when a nerve cell is close enough to excite a neighboring nerve cell, changes occur in the communication and connectivity of these nerve cells. If a particular neural activation pattern persists and continues to be reinforced, the connections become stronger and more efficient.[84] This theory eventually birthed the catchy neuroscience rhyme, "Nerves that fire together wire together." (A big thanks to neurobiologist, Carla Shatz for this one!) In other words, the more an activity or behavior is repeated, the stronger the neural connections and associated patterns.

The brain adapts with all experiences and recruits multiple brain areas for predictive coding and long-term memory. We know that the pain experience (acute or chronic) is not always directly correlated to tissue damage. However, when pain persists, it becomes *decreasingly* related to the actual state of the tissues. In other words, pain is an unpleasant sensory and emotional experience, but the longer it goes on, changes take place in our physiology that may make the emotional part of the pain experience stronger. As such, areas of the brain that are involved with learning and emotions also intermingle with the neurological pathways involved in our experience of pain.[85] Memories are also strengthened the more you recall and think about them. This process of *learning* in the pain experience changes neuron structure, and neurons become more efficient at firing in a particular pattern.

Thankfully, with some clever retraining, you can change pain by establishing a new relationship with it, finding opportunities that reinforce safe and positive experiences with your body and mind. Before you know it, you'll be sprouting new neuronal pathways that will eventually outgrow the old ones.[86]

Your brain always wants to know what's going on, so it's only natural for danger sensors in your tissues, and your nerve and immune cells in your brain and spinal cord to alter and adapt, sometimes recruiting other neighboring areas to join in on the conversation; this means your pain might feel like it's playing tricks on you. First it's here, then it's there, jumping around all over the place. This is actually another good indication that pain is most likely due to a sensitive and protective nervous system and not tissue damage. Feeling muscle tension and tightness is a common protective response to a 'perceived' threat, but that doesn't necessarily mean being directly in harm's way. If someone jokes around pretending they're going to hit you in the nads, you're going to brace or jump regardless of whether they touch you or not. Again, a very natural and normal response to have.

My advice here is try a new mantra: "I'm sore, but I'm safe." (Another shout out to Dr. David Butler for this one).

THOUGHTS AND THE VICIOUS CYCLE OF CATASTROPHIZING

Ever heard a voice in your head telling you something like: *this pain's never going to go away*? You're not alone. Distressing thoughts and worry can run rampant through your head when you've got persistent pain. This is a normal human thing too! What you might not know is that believing in everything your mind tells you about your pain might be holding you back from flourishing in life. I say this knowing very well that it's not easy to feel at peace with these thoughts, but it is possible to pull back the reins on your mind.

As we've already touched on, pain can worsen just by thinking about a perceived threat via actual neurophysiological responses. You've watched a horror movie, right? Remember the escape scene from *The Silence of the Lambs*, for example, where Hannibal Lecter bites off the prison guard's face? I'm willing to bet you knew what was coming. Didn't it make your heart beat just a little quicker and your muscles tense up? The reason I mention this is to show you how you don't have to be in any actual direct danger for your brain to interpret it as such, causing your body to physiologically respond in a protective way and your behavior to change. You'll feel real emotions and feelings watching pixels on a screen even though you know it isn't real. The *potential* threat alone can create a pain sensation without any actual tissue damage or injury.

If horror movies aren't your thing, how about this story? I once asked my husband if he or his friends had ever performed self-inflicted torture to their testicles, just mucking around. He remembered a time when he and his buddy messed about with what they thought was an unloaded BB gun, shooting each other with air at close range. His friend Mike thought it would be a fun idea to test out the gun at close range, pointing the gun to his balls. Unfortunately, it wasn't just air that came out that time. Mike didn't know it, but a BB had fallen into the chamber. One black and blue ball later, Mike was jumping around with tears in his eyes at the horrific pain that followed. Did you just make your *oh-shit-that's-gotta-hurt* face when reading that? Maybe even felt the urge to protect your own family jewels? That's your body's response to just reading and imagining a not-so-fun situation. The thought of a BB gun shooting you in the nads makes you flinch and protect them. Get where I'm going with this?

Pain is both a protective response and a sensory experience in your body like overly sensitive touch or movement or feelings of anxiety from the stress dealing with pain. Your thoughts and beliefs about pain can be liberating, or they can perpetuate more anxiety. Depends on your perspective.

Are you willing to try something with me? If you said yes, go ahead and grab a letter-sized piece of paper. Let's pretend your pain thoughts,

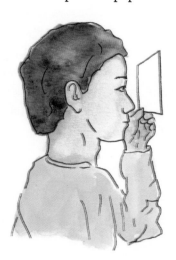

struggles, and frustrations are represented by this piece of paper and everything outside the of this piece of paper represents what's most important to you in life.[87]

Now place the piece of paper close to your nose, like in the image on page 48.

What do you see?

Next, move the piece of paper an arm's length away.

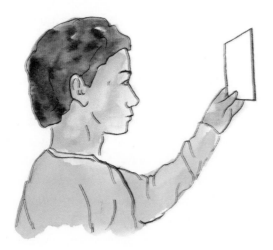

Now, what do you see?

This can be translated to your pain experience. The pain didn't go away, but you see the world differently. Now imagine what life would be like holding this piece of paper in your hand 24/7 while doing things like driving, making dinner, or having sex. Life would be challenging, wouldn't it? (For one, papercuts would be a major buzz kill.) So, what would happen if you set the piece of paper down right next to you? The pain is still there, but life just got a bit easier to navigate. Just like you did with the piece of paper, if pain is making your world look small, what can you do to expand your view and make life bigger?

There's a storm brewing. You can watch this storm from two

perspectives: standing behind the window pane or standing outside getting soaking wet. Which experience would you prefer to have during the storm? Either way, it's happening. The longer and more persistently distressing thoughts loop around in your mind, the more the nervous system will adapt and amp up stronger, more powerful ways to protect you. Eventually, other neighboring neurons corresponding to different parts of your virtual body map in the brain will also start getting in on the action, even though that part of your body is completely healthy. You could say *guilty by association.*

Immobilizing fear and perpetually distressing thoughts are strong predictors that your central nervous system is ramped up.[88] Researchers discovered that the combination of long-standing pelvic pain with un-relenting worrisome thoughts actually changes the brain structure and function over time.[89] [90] [91] The front left part of your brain deals with positive feelings like hope and joy. The front right part of your brain deals with emotions like anxiety and sadness. Scientists noticed that those who have persistent pain have reduced activity in the left part of the brain and increased activity in the right. That means feeling more down in the dumps, socially withdrawn and hopeless when long-standing pain combines with the distressing thought behavior already mentioned.

Stress and anxiety (such as that related to persistent pain) also influence your brain structure and function, which in turn impacts how your penis functions. Mental stress activates physiological, chemical and behavioral changes all at the same time.[92] Feelings such as pleasure and pain are conscious snapshots of our perceived sense of wellbeing. They are like a report card grading our psychological and biological equilibrium.[93] [94] Dr. Antonio Damasio, a neuroscientist whose research focuses on feelings, emotions, and consciousness, would argue that feelings are not the same as emotions. Emotions have been described as neurophysiological phenomena in response to inner and outer world information, including our sensory experiences. Feelings, on the other hand, are personal judgments (good, bad; pleasant, unpleasant) of our experiences and their consequences. Feelings also serve to help us learn from these experiences in anticipation of potentially beneficial or harmful future situations. Emotions and their relative feelings influence cellular processes, learning, motivation, drive, behavior, habits, and reactions to life events both at an individual and sociocultural level.[95] Emotions might also represent what's happening at the organ level and vice versa. For example, have you ever felt embarrassed and noticed your face get red? That's an example of these physiological changes that occur in response to certain states of being that translate to a conscious and highly subjective mental experience (AKA feelings). Emotions and feelings are interconnected, and the deeper, older parts of our brain and gut play an important role in our experience of those feelings. These same structures also play an important role in our experience of pain and pleasure. The pain you experience around loss when you're going through a break-up and the pain you experience from slicing your thumb cutting vegetables is physiologically expressed in the same way. In other words, both painful experiences are similar in the way they happen in the body biologically.

Pain (physical or emotional) is a feeling that motivates us to take action in relation to our body and to our life. It urges us to pay attention and reflect on our whole life. It signals 'something's gotta give,' because if you continue on the same path, it might not turn out well. Here's the caveat: not all emotions are translated into a mental experience as a feeling. Feelings, especially negative ones, that do arise are mental experiences of mind that might lead to suffering depending on our point of view.

In cases of pain, not all aches and pains lead to suffering. For example, if you stub your toe, does it hurt? Yes. For how long? Most likely just a few seconds or minutes. Do you suffer as a result? Not really. Why? Because you've probably stubbed your toe in the past, know the feeling and can understand exactly what happened to your toe because you can see it. Your dick hurting is another story. You can't show your friends, you've never experienced this kind of sensation in your pleasure bits before, and you can't really see *why* you hurt or understand the cause. For these very reasons, the problem in your pants gradually grows more and more unpleasant, resulting in *suffering*. Pain isn't the problem here, it's the 'putting life on hold' part that often trips people up.

And if your thoughts, behaviors, past experiences, stress, and fears continue to haunt you, it's no wonder your brain keeps signaling to you that your private parts are in danger. Naturally, your muscles tense up, get tighter and impact the overall health and perception of your genitals and their function.

The replaying of events – ahem, like the frustrations of having to deal with pelvic pain – also activate similar brain areas, further driving your stress response. What if you could do like the pro tennis players do and let the match point go? I know, it's simple, but not easy. Like learning a new skill, this way of thinking and being takes a lot practice.

The purpose of telling you all this is to help you understand the miraculous and amazing processes involved in the human body that allow you to sense the world you live in, which is uniquely experienced by each individual. Just like a thumb print, no two are ever the same. So, if you come across messages that blame pain on your posture, your alignment, your muscles, or your stressed-out state, now you'll have the knowledge to understand that pain is more complex than that. Many of the things that get 'blamed' for persistent pain are not biologically plausible and have even been disputed by the current evidence. It's oh-so-much more complex. Many people in pain have found that when they stop chasing pain and take a break from resisting it and forcing it to go away, they find greater ease and more success. Would you be willing to take a break from chasing pain? What does it feel like when you ask yourself to consider stop looking for the why?

Now, I hope you're not thinking that you're shit up a creek without a paddle! Just as your body has some pretty clever ways to protect you, it also has the ability to turn pain into pleasure. If you don't believe me, just ask former Red Hot Chili Peppers guitarist Dave Navarro. Dave likes to hang his body from hooks to relax. *The Guardian* quoted Dave saying, "Sometimes it's just fun, but it can also be very meditative. If I've been in a deep depression for a few weeks, a few hooks and a few feet in the air and I'm feeling radiant and optimistic again."[96]

Don't go hanging yourself from hooks just yet! There are many other ways to go pleasure-hunting to help retrain your brain. One of these ways is tapping into the 'drug cabinet' in your brain by purposefully searching for, creating and building on novel, positive experiences related to the bits that hurt and elsewhere, not just in your body but

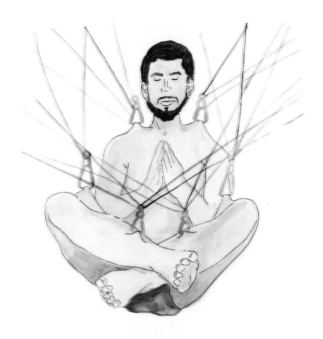

also your life. Doing this activates areas of the brain associated with the 'reward system' and pleasure. These areas light up during activities like meditation, doing something you enjoy, having fun with friends, watching a funny movie, or stimulating your taste buds with something yummy. These areas, when lit, have the opposite effect on your threat detection systems, decreasing distress, fear, and the need for protection. I just love science, don't you?

Physical and emotional stress has been shown to make concentration and everyday function exhausting. No wonder pelvic pain can be draining and make you so tired all the time. The energy and attention you give to your pain is tiring you out, especially since thoughts are actual physical nerve impulses.

But if your thoughts and beliefs have the ability to influence pain, they also have the ability to help you out of pain. Which is the good news. Enter the autonomic nervous system, your body's regulator.

GETTING ON YOUR NERVES

From the nerve anatomy section in the last chapter, you may have figured out already that your nerves are important because they make up the communication highway between the body and the brain. The central nervous system is what I like to call the 'big boss,' and this boss works two shifts: 'rest and digest' and 'fight, flight, or freeze.' These two states collectively make up your autonomic nervous system (ANS), which is responsible for regulating your bodily functions, communicating with your brain and organs, responding to emergency and non-emergency situations. There's also the *enteric nervous system*, but we'll get into that when we talk about gut health.

In the case of pelvic pain, there usually isn't a mechanism of injury to blame. The onset is rather ambiguous. Typically if there's been an injury, healing times will vary depending on the type of tissue involved, severity of the injury, and your overall state of health. Healing time may range from a few days to several months.[97] [98] [99] Once tissues have healed, any persisting symptoms are less likely attributed to tissue injury. There are other mechanisms at play that we need to investigate, namely, the collection of processes encompassing the biological, psychological and sociological aspects of your pain experience. Ruminating and distressing thoughts in your head have an impact on your feeling and experience of pain.

Think you're maybe dealing with more than just a muscle issue here? Study your thoughts, as they should tip you off. Some thoughts that indicate your mind and edgy nervous system are in play with your pain could include:

I keep thinking about how much it hurts.
My life is ruined.
It's hard to stay focused on a single task.
I'll never get rid of this.
I can't sleep.
My digestive system is wonky.
The pain keeps moving around.
Nothing helps anymore.

My pain gets worse when I'm stressed or anxious.
The pain comes out of nowhere.
Places that never used to hurt now hurt.
The pills don't even work. I don't know why I'm taking them.
I'm afraid the pain will get worse.
I'm more forgetful these days.

Can you relate to any of those statements? Maybe you've even used some of them in the past? Statements like these are indicators that the pain is probably not coming from your tissues. It's got more to do with your threat detection systems and the central nervous system (although what's happening at the nerve endings in your tissues can also play a role). Of the two 'states' I identified as making up the central nervous system, the *sympathetic nervous system* is your 'fight, flight, or freeze' response mechanism. The Mike Tyson of the nerve world, it's the switch that quickly turns on when you need protection or when you're getting ready to jump out of a plane skydiving with your friends.

Adrenaline, norepinephrine, and cortisol are stress hormones that help protect you. When this fight or flight switch is turned on, your body gets flooded with stress hormones so your gut gets sluggish (no time to spend energy on digesting food right now), your heart and respiratory rate increase, you sweat bullets, get goosebumps, your energy and power are amped up, you become super motivated to take action, and your brain makes sure you don't have the urge to poop, pee, or feel aroused while fighting for your life (because that would be bad). Neurohormones (hormones that act like chemical messengers) are released from your brain and adrenal glands (in both pain and non-pain situations) and influence the areas of the brain that modulate fear and other emotions, thus impacting the fear-based stress response mechanisms throughout your entire body.[100]

These are all important reactions when you're actually in danger, but what happens when your body goes through this on a daily basis via physical and psychological stressors? When you don't come down from that high-stress rollercoaster ride? When you don't know when your next flare-up is going to be? When you still have no clue why you're in pain?

Pain in itself is a major stressor, and anything that threatens your tissues, your personhood or your existence will activate physiological stress response mechanisms to protect you. If the threat in your undercarriage doesn't get extinguished early on, these stress response mechanisms can become overly sensitive to any potential and/or actual noxious stimuli and further solidify this pain memory pattern (especially since it has to do with the most intimate parts of your body) eliciting protection with even non-threatening stimuli.[101] Cortisol has also been said to promote the efficiency and growth of neural connections in the amygdala, which further strengthens the fear associated with negative experiences such as pain.[102] The consolidation of a memory is what's called a 'distributed process' across the brain, meaning several areas across the brain communicate, influence each other, and light up at the same time, including the spinal cord, nerve endings in tissues and immune system.

The stress response mechanisms are *just one* of the many, many processes involved in this complicated orchestra of events. Pain-related or not, there can be many other triggers activating and reinforcing a predicted outcome of pain... Case in point: those forums you find yourself scouring for hours on end! Anything that reinforces this negative, unpleasant experience and expectation will impact how you feel and how your body responds to this stressor.[103] This includes:

➤ Failed treatments
➤ What others have told you about your pain
➤ What you read on the internet
➤ Prior experiences with pain
➤ Observation of other people's 'bad' outcomes
➤ Your expectations and general outlook on the situation
➤ Thoughts and beliefs
➤ Avoidance of activities where pain is anticipated

The consequences of a nervous system gone haywire are a sympathetic overload and the release of chemical messengers by way of hormones like adrenaline, norepinephrine and cortisol. Over time, this 'fight or flight' chemical release can affect your immunity, the ability to heal and repair tissues, concentration, cognitive function, mood, muscle tone, blood pressure, hormonal function, sleep patterns, digestive system, libido and brain structure... Just to name a few.[104]

Wait a sec?! Did I just suggest a loss in libido from stress?! Yup, I sure did. Cortisol, one of the stress hormones, acts as a protector in many ways. In acute situations, cortisol helps ward off inflammation in the body, for one. However, under longer bouts of stress, the immune system gets riled up as normal stress response mechanisms become altered (cortisol no longer keeping the immune cells in check). Some people might experience an underproduction of cortisol and other people might experience an overproduction of cortisol. It all depends on the individual, the context of the situation and the environmental factors at play. Typically, persisting pain will result in impaired stress response mechanisms, although the ongoing pain itself can contribute to this altered process. You might be wondering what this mechanism has to do with pain in the pelvis. It's been well-documented that men with persistent pelvic pain (and those who experience ongoing pain elsewhere in their body) have altered stress response mechanisms and neuroimmune function.[105] [106]

Speaking of inflammation, it's not the *only* trigger for pain or tissue issues. Inflammation can be helpful and not so helpful; it depends on the context. In fact, when you sprain your ankle, we want inflammation! It's an indicator of tissue healing. Furthermore, inflammation might be present, but that still doesn't mean you'll experience any symptoms. As an example, if men with and without pelvic pain have similar results when white blood cells in urine and prostatic fluid are compared, perhaps the reliability of these diagnostic biomarkers should be taken with a grain of salt.[107] In other words, biomarkers, like in a lot of other syndromes, are not 100% reliable or indicative of the cause for pain. This is even recognized by the NIH. Remember their fourth classification of prostatitis? Asymptomatic inflammatory prostatitis. Go figure!

You'll be happy to hear that for all there is a Mike Tyson of the nerve world, there is also a Mahatma Gandhi. The *parasympathetic nervous system* is the 'rest and digest' response system. When this switch is turned on, it lets you digest that meal you just ate, relaxes your heart rate and breathing, stimulates the production of calming chemical messengers like serotonin (the 'happy' chemical of the brain that is produced mostly in your gut), relaxes your muscles, and allows your bladder and bowel to relax so that you can take care of business.

When your body is unable to come back down from an overly aroused nervous system, it begins to work on overdrive, which can exacerbate your current pain experience. Whenever you find yourself 'freaking out' or feeling a lack of control in any situation, this will dial up the alarm system and intensify your pain experience. When your body is in homeostasis (the happy place between the two extremes of the nervous systems); however, it has the ability to heal itself as well as stimulate normal bodily functions in order for you to combat the demands of life, including sex. Woohoo! Now we're getting somewhere.

Let's get real here; stress in life is unavoidable. The good news is, you have some control over what you perceive as stressful and how you respond to it. This is a gentle reminder that there's hope for your pain to change. There are possibilities where there used to be little or none. Yet again, I'm driving the point here that how you think about your pain can influence the physiological processes underpinning ongoing perpetuation of pain.

EFFECTS OF PROLONGED PAIN AND STRESS ON OTHER SYSTEMS

Of course, it's a little more complex than just positive-thinking and resting, because it's not just the nervous system at play. (It's all connected, remember!) There are multiple body systems that all work together to protect you so that you can function at your best. They're constantly communicating and were designed so that, if one system is underperforming for some reason, another one has to take up the slack.

Persistent pain can affect any of these systems (and vice versa):
➤ Urinary
➤ Reproductive
➤ Skeletal
➤ Endocrine
➤ Immune
➤ Nervous

➤ Respiratory
➤ Muscular
➤ Cardiovascular
➤ Lymphatic
➤ Digestive

As we've seen in the last section, when you're physically or emotionally stressed, your body activates that 'fight or flight' response in the nervous system to protect you. Multiple systems are involved when it comes to protecting you from a perceived or actual threat. The effect of this on other systems is worth noting.

Let's revisit the immune system. As you've already learned, under prolonged stress, your cells receive a signal to promote inflammation. Again, not a bad thing in the short term, but with impaired function, eventually cortisol catches up and doesn't counteract this inflammatory state. As such, chemical changes can affect your immune system by producing more inflammatory chemical messengers and at times autoimmunity against even healthy tissues. This can even 'wake up' old aches and pains just by tapping into the neuroimmune system's memory bank. Have you ever had the flu? I bet you probably ached all over. This is your wonderful immune system at work, the policemen of your body aiding repair and restoration. Along with a cellular pro-inflammatory state comes the depletion of serotonin, the 'happy' neurotransmitter, too. No wonder you're not in the mood… for anything!

And what about the muscular system? You won't be surprised that, as always, this is all connected and related, too. The muscular system doesn't get let off the hook when we're talking about prolonged stress, either. Prolonged cellular stress and damage can cause tissues in your body to become unhealthy and diminish your ability to heal and repair. It's no coincidence that we call stressed-out, controlling people 'uptight' or 'anal retentive.' When you're under stress, a bit anxious, tired but wired, your pelvic floor might respond in the same way.

Recognizing when and where you hold tension in your body is key to start letting it go. Go ahead and make a fist with your hand. Squeeze it really hard, then let go. If you can turn up tension, you can turn it down too. If you haven't figured it out already, your emotions and intentions affect your motor function, including muscle tension and ability to relax, because the body and the mind are so intimately connected.

A research study from 2001 showed the relationship between stress and pelvic muscle tension in women. (Sorry guys, I couldn't find one specific to male bodies, but stay with me!) The women in the study were exposed to threatening and non-threatening video clips while vaginal sensors recorded muscle activity. Researchers found that pelvic muscles responded to the threatening stimuli before the women could take conscious action as a defensive mechanism.[108] In other words, when safety is at stake, these muscles go into protective mode automatically. Remember our bruise-balled friend Mike? Just reading about his story probably made you tense down there, right?

When you're under stress, you start unconsciously developing 'holding patterns' or tension within the body. For you, maybe it so happens to be in the pelvic floor. Now don't get me wrong, having tension in muscles doesn't necessarily mean you're doomed to have pain for the rest of your life. There are many people who have tight muscles and experience no pain. Tension is not to blame.

Persistent or prolonged holding patterns may lead to altered pelvic muscle function and altered tissue health, which might even contribute to changes in bowel and bladder function. After a while, your body might get cranky, compensating for this imbalance in your body and in your life, and will let you know, like "Hello, I'm talking to you," AKA pain. If ignored long enough, this message might get louder and louder, until it's screaming bloody murder to get your attention. If this was your hamstring muscle, for example, you probably wouldn't think much about it, but it's your penis we're talking about, so naturally tensions start to rise (and not in a good way).

On it goes... Louder and louder... Creating more anxiety, more pain, more anxiety, more pain. This perpetuating fear can trap you in a vicious pain-tension cycle. Just another example of how your thoughts can influence pain. (So you know, using WebMD to self-diagnose isn't the smartest idea if you want to get out of this anxiety trap.)

The vicious circle goes round and round until you decide it's time to get off. Unrelenting anxiety and worry feed the pro-inflammatory cascade and will increase those stress chemical messengers to your brain (and tissues), which can then alter neuroimmune thresholds, increasing your sensitivity. It's kinda like a smoke alarm that goes off when all you do is blow on it. The damn thing goes blaring, but there's nothing serious going on. The problem with alarms is they're designed to be sensitive. Just like your fight or flight response. Everyone's alarms are designed differently.

But just as I've mentioned previously and want to reiterate here and now, your pain isn't permanent. If you can turn it up, you can turn it down, sorta like a volume dial. Even though your outer problems may seem endless, your inner problems are solvable.

So, what's the first step to getting a handle on your mental and physical tension? Becoming aware of it. It's sometimes hard (and scary) to bring awareness inside your body and inside your head when you've been so distracted by the outside, especially by all the things done to avoid, get rid of and control pain. What does it take to come back home to your body and get back to your life? Mental flexibility, mental resilience, practice, patience, acceptance and an understanding that you can't 'control' external circumstances no matter how hard you try, because things change and life happens however much we plan.

Do you find your mind is often tight, agitated, frustrated, angry, or in victim mode whenever things don't go your way or you can't control outcomes or external circumstances? If so, you may end up rarely feeling satisfied or pleased with treatment outcomes or in life. Often, the more attached we are to the outcome, the more disappointed we become when things don't go the way we want.

Breaking the pain-guarding-tension-anxiety cycle is possible. It takes patience, practice, commitment, and some TLC with loads of self-compassion. Compassion is the feeling you get when you recognize suffering in others and allow their experience to touch you deeply. In that moment, it moves you to make space in your heart for their suffering and pain. Instead of ignoring them, judging them, or hardening your heart, it softens with a motivation to help them in some way. Self-compassion is similar in that we give ourselves permission to open up and soften our heart to our own struggles and suffering. When we accept our own suffering compassionately, we can become a source of refuge for others. In what ways could you use your experience with pain to deepen compassion for yourself and others? To test your self-compassion, visit: www.self-compassion.org/test-how-self-compassionate-you-are/

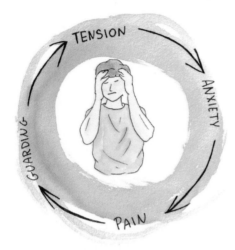

The remainder of this book is dedicated to the process of owning your pain, embracing a different relationship with your body, and going easy on yourself as you embark on this journey. If you let go of worry, expectations and anxieties about getting better, you'll be surprised how much easier it will be to navigate through pelvic pain. It's like holding onto the end of a rope that just keeps getting tugged on. The harder you hold on to that rope, the more it hurts. What if you considered letting go of the rope? Do you think that could provide a chance to make the struggle a bit easier? How does it feel when you entertain that thought?

Before you get the idea that I'm saying your pain is all in your head, please know that's not what this is about. Your pain is real, you physically feel it in your body, and you want it to go away. I understand that. However, all this science points to an absolutely key piece of knowledge that can unlock a better path forward: a peaceful mind is more helpful to feeling better than an angry, despondent, or agitated mind.

The fact that you're dealing with this pain is not your choice, but you do have a choice in how you respond to the adversities that come your way.

CHAPTER 4

MAKING YOUR MIND UP

Athlete Michael Phelps wouldn't have won 28 career Olympic medals without challenging and working on his mindset.[109] Many athletes train with sports psychologists to "overcome mental roadblocks and improve their performance."[110] There are many different ways to train your mental muscle, and like everything else, there is no one-size-fits-all solution. Some familiar approaches may include a combination of mental rehearsing, somatic therapy, cognitive behavioral therapy, acceptance and commitment therapy, and mindfulness-based stress reduction strategies. These psychologically informed strategies offer an opportunity to explore the relationship we have with our internal experiences, such as pain, rather than trying to change the experience itself. Recognizing thoughts and feelings that get in the way of living your best life will uncover choices rather than ultimatums, assuming that you're willing to experience all that life has to offer no matter how pleasant or painful these experiences might be. Embracing this mission will move you closer towards living a life chock-full of purpose and meaning. So, are you willing to rethink your relationship with pain?

It's not uncommon for men with pelvic pain to feel hopeless, angry, depressed and frustrated about their symptoms. In fact, anxiety and depression usually go hand in hand with men who experience pelvic pain and is one of the factors that might contribute to the chronicity of pain.[111] And who could blame you if you're feeling this way? We're talking about your manhood, the one thing that (at least according to pretty much everything men get told by society) defines your masculinity. Problems with the plumbing would make anyone worried and anxious. But what happens when these thoughts rattle around in your brain longer than you'd like? Repetitive attention to thoughts like, 'I'll never get better,' 'It's ruined my life,' 'I'll live like this for the rest of my life' or 'My life revolves around pelvic pain' light up pain *neurotags* (collection of neurons in the brain that fire together) making the pathway activate more efficiently and stronger the next time it's activated.

Our mind's job is to think and problem-solve. Without awareness, we might haphazardly follow what our mind tells us. However, when you begin to notice your thoughts, you have an opportunity to make choices in your life that either move you towards or away from things in life that are important to you instead of being ruled by your thoughts.

Going to see a mental health professional can sometimes be stigmatized because of the way society views men in relation to their feelings. So, if it helps to think about this as mental coaching, know that plenty of people have this useful addition on their wellness team. It's about training your brain to find a different path, a path of least resistance, one that liberates your mind and doesn't take life too seriously, just like the pros do.

OWNING YOUR PELVIC PAIN

Let's start with the first helpful mind trick to tackle your pelvic pain: owning it. Now, nobody wants to 'own' their pelvic pain or any pain for that matter, but there's some truth to the benefits behind why you should. Pelvic pain doesn't happen overnight. It might seem like it did. Yet in most cases, it's a build-up of events, causes and conditions coming together to create the perfect storm. This triggers the body to make a screeching halt and say, 'Hey, pay attention to me!' It's your body telling you that something has to change, whether that's lifestyle, thoughts, behaviors, or your annoying boss. (Yep, seriously!) Sometimes it's not that easy to change your outer world, and even if you could change some things, this isn't a guarantee for fixing your inner world experience, including pain. So, when pain shows up in your life, how do you handle it?

The body is constantly trying to adjust and adapt to the daily grind that it goes through. Some people are better than others at finding that 'life balance.' But it's okay if you're not one of them. Just like you can beef up your biceps, you can also strengthen your mental flexibility by shifting your focus and attention to what matters most to you in life.

In conventional medicine, the approach is more biomedical, a 'find it and fix it' mentality, which means you tend to outsource responsibility and power for your health. Healthcare providers are guides. They provide education and potential options to help you through a health challenge, but they can't 'fix' the inner experience of pain. They can only help with biological underpinnings that may be contributing and sometimes find a temporary resolution. Putting your hopes of success in someone else's hands makes you a greater target for disappointment, frustration, anger, or blame. Yet, dealing with an 'invisible' condition is indeed daunting and scary. Men with CP/CPPS don't tend to feel validated and are often dismissed by healthcare providers. CPPS is a diagnosis of exclusion, which means that there isn't a clear-cut answer to explain why there's pain down there. This also means that many invasive tests and procedures are done before this conclusion is even made, which can add to the frustration, fear, hopelessness and ongoing pain. Men with CP/CPPS compare their quality of life to patients who have had a heart attack, Crohn's disease or diabetes.[112]

Painful sensations and emotions are not often the cause for our suffering; it's the unrelenting and insatiable quest to avoid, change, and control these unpleasant feelings that forces us to put life on hold. We've all had the thought: *I'll get back to <fill in your blank> once this problem goes away.* If you're feeling this way, it's a normal story to hear about pelvic pain. Indeed, Nicholas Wood and his colleagues wrote a paper reflecting the stories and experiences of 12 men living with pelvic pain. The authors summarized three common threads:[113]

1) *Blame and shame* – Lack of support and validation, negative medical interactions, and many invasive tests and treatments with limited success.

2) *Rollercoaster ride* – Symptoms are often unpredictable, or come and go. It is hard to find triggers, which makes every situation an uncertain one. There's a sense of lack of control over your life, body, and behavior.

3) *Ongoing struggle for coping and cures* – One of the main struggles is not having an outlet or space to talk about your experience or feelings. There are sociocultural stigmas around 'being a man' and 'manning up'. There's also a deep desire to find the 'magic cure', only to be left more frustrated and hopeless. Life gets consumed with activities around trying to control or avoid pain, which often leads you to put life on hold.

Strategies that helped this particular group of men included staying positive, being active, utilizing support, and finding meaning and purpose for their pain experience.

People in pain want to know:

➤ Why do I hurt?
➤ How long will it take to get better?
➤ What can I do to help myself?
➤ What can others do to help me?

These are all valid and reasonable questions to ask. The 'how long?' question is probably on the forefront of your mind. When we know there's an end in sight, enduring temporary discomfort doesn't seem so bad. We can all endure discomfort and pain knowing that it will end at some point. The problem is that with persistent pain, there's a lot of uncertainty. Every day is unpredictable, and this in itself keeps the threat detection systems on high alert. Secondly, although there might not be a single known cause to explain why you hurt, I hope this book has provided you with pieces of knowledge to put your puzzle together and make sense of it all. Life is a process to be lived, not a problem to be solved.

Completely relying on others to 'fix' you might lead you to a dead end. We try to 'fix' a problem by holding on to it tightly, and ruminating about it over and over again. How do you 'fix' an internal problem like pain with external solutions? Take a moment to reflect on your own experience dealing with pelvic pain. What have you done to avoid, control or get rid of pain? Where did it lead you? What does your experience tell you? This isn't to say that we don't seek support and guidance from others, because anything we can do to shift the pain narrative and get 'unstuck' is a pivot towards engaging in a life of purpose and meaning. As Buddhist monk Shantideva once said, "Suffering has many great qualities."[114]

If pain plans to stick around for an uncertain amount of time, how *could* you work with it? Although not instantly gratifying, exploring pain in this way might allow you to shift into new perspectives on your situation. When we allow ourselves to hang out with discomfort, anger, frustration and pain, we start to become curious, courageous, and deepen our compassion for ourselves and others. As a result, a seed of calmness will sprout. It's knowing that no matter how much the situation sucks right now, everything will be okay.

This is why owning your pain is the first step to taking back control. It means more working in and less working out. And it's a huge shift in mindset that's going to help change how you relate to your current predicament. So… it's okay to own it!

BUT WHY ME?

As worrying as it is to have pelvic pain, you could and should take it one step further and even be thankful for it. *Whaaa?!* You read that right. Let's thank your body and mind for giving you the heads-up that something's gotta change. It's the subtle hints we forget to pay attention to that lead up to a major wakeup call like pelvic pain. Our body (and mind) gives out warning signs to nudge us to listen more closely to our needs so we can respond to them, so we can protect ourselves from continuing down a path that wouldn't lead to a happy ending (if you catch my drift). In such a busy world, those signals often get lost in the crowd.

Taking care of yourself isn't just about a healthy diet and exercising, because let's face it, even some of the craziest health nuts I know get sick, including me. Sometimes there's no rhyme or reason. It just happens. Life just happens. We need to leave some wiggle room for uncertainty. The more space we can reserve for uncertainty, the less of a blow we'll feel when certain circumstances in life sideswipe us. We all have our 'moments.' It's a shared human experience, just like pain. If you've ever watched surfers, you know that they embrace the wipeouts (hell, I think they even enjoy it). They'll lose their surf board, pull it back and get right back on to catch the next wave. No matter how big or small, how calm or turbulent, waves are still just waves, and learning to 'ride the wave' with humility, persistence and mental flexibility will allow you to persevere even in the face of unrelenting adversity.

Dr. Lissa Rankin, MD asks her patients two questions during their appointment: "What do you think might lie at the root of your illness?" and "What does your body need in order to heal?" You might say something like, "I need to lose weight," "I need to exercise more," or "I have to stop eating donuts for breakfast," but most of the time it's the elephant in the room that you avoid at all costs, like, "I hate my job," "I'm not in love with my partner anymore," "I need a break," "I hate where I live," "I don't know what to do with my life," "I need more fun," "I don't have friends," and so on and so on. Your thoughts and emotions both impact and reflect the story of your insides and the reality of your world. I love the way Dr. Rankin puts it, "The body doesn't fuel how we live our lives. Instead, it is a mirror of how we live our lives."[115]

So, I challenge you right now to ask yourself those two questions. *What do I think is perpetuating my pain? What does my body need in order for it to feel well?* It's okay if you don't have the answers right away. Remember, navigating pelvic pain is a journey, and discovering the answer to these questions might be part of the quest.

SHHH, BE QUIET!

Quieting down an upregulated nervous system takes time, patience, commitment, and some brain-y tricks. Imagine walking around with your biceps flexed as if you were showing off your guns for two years straight. How do you think that arm will start feeling? After one day? A month? A year? Okay, I'm exaggerating the point, but it's to explain what happens to the pelvic floor muscles when protective mechanisms kick into gear. It's sorta like an overprotective parent. You've got to prove that you're safe to play on the playground without getting hurt. The muscles might adapt to function differently, and the vascular system, nerves and organs (including your brain) start to adapt to the new situation, too. A friendly reminder: although these changes occur, they are not permanent. Things can get better. You can change.

You probably weren't even aware that your pelvic muscles existed until things went awry. And that's the thing. It's likely that there was a lack of body awareness and intuition over a long period, so the subtle messages of your body were ignored. And who's to blame you? When things are working alright down there, you shouldn't be thinking about your pelvic muscles just like you don't think about your food being digested. But to some extent, there's an underlying sense of self that you can pick up on if you're willing to listen.

So, first things first. Let's get quiet enough to know what your body feels like on a subtle level, rather than just fixating on the pain. Right now, pain is fighting for the TV remote, jumping all over your lap, trying to dictate your movie selection. It's pretty obnoxious. But here's the thing, it's not going away. So, you can do one of two things: lock it outside, hoping it just goes away or make space for this pestering friend to sit right beside you on the couch. The first approach just makes the pain scream louder, banging on the door to come back in, which doesn't make for happy neighbors. However, the second option creates some space between you and the pain so that you can let go of the struggle (just a little), breathe a little easier, all the while continuing to help yourself move towards a happier, more fulfilling life, even with your newfound friend.

Now, don't get me wrong. Making friends with pain might feel a bit weird. It's perfectly normal to feel uncomfortable in your own skin during this process of letting go. We all go through 'growing pains' when our cells start to change. It's called *resistance*. Whenever you're trying to change a behavior, habit, or whatever else, there's a process that your mind and body go through. It's like that New Year's resolution you set for yourself. "I'm going to exercise every day for an hour." Okay great! So, January 1st rolls around and you're pumped, ready to take action and rock 'n' roll. The first week you're amped and proud that you've stuck with it for a whole seven days. As soon as that second week hits, it feels like such a drag. Then come the excuses and you're back to where you were last year. Sound familiar? Does for me. Your brain and cells actually go through physical and chemical changes when you're learning a new behavior or transforming an old one. To paraphrase W. Clement Stone, "Small hinges swing open large doors." In other words, even the smallest of changes add up to really big transformations. It's sticking with it and trusting the process even when there appears to be evidence to the contrary. Change is hard for anyone, and learning to down-train overly hyped-up 'everything' takes grit.

And did I already mention patience...?

BUT I WANT IT NOW

So, how much time will this take? To be honest, I don't know. I don't think anyone can whip out a crystal ball and tell you either. (And if they do, run!) Everyone's situation is different, and the time it takes to recover will vary based on your unique set of circumstances and individual needs. That being said – and I know you might not want to hear this – we need to have a heart-to-heart conversation over here. We need to leave on the table the possibility that pain might be in the background... for an indefinite amount of time. Pelvic pain didn't happen overnight, and it won't go away overnight either. I know this is a hard concept to grasp in a world where instant gratification prevails and you've got answers just seconds away in the palm of your hands. Yet change really does require daily practice and attention to your overall needs. Your perspective contributes greatly to this process. You can be in the driver's seat, or you can be the passenger. In other words, you can choose to have pain dictate your life, or you can take the bull by its horns and get back to living. Remember, your thoughts and emotions trigger actual physical reactions that keep you riding the pain merry-go-round.

The harder you try to get rid of the pain, the more push-back you'll get. Trying equals effort, and effort equals work. But it's not the trying that's the issue here. It's *how* you do the trying, *how* you show up, and what kind of mind you have during the process. It's one thing to do an exercise, a stretch, or meditation just for the sake of doing it, but are you truly present without grasping to the outcome tightly? Having a balanced mind, a mind that is okay with whatever arises, makes navigating through difficult situations just a teeny-tiny bit lighter. Acceptance, self-compassion, and understanding that you're not alone in this struggle will keep the tension, stress, and anxiety at bay, allowing your body to take the lead and recover.

Your body is a miracle (heck, your life is a miracle if you really think about it) and has the intrinsic ability to transform and adapt in some pretty amazing ways. You just have to trust it. A life without pain is possible.

TEMPER TANTRUMS AWAIT

What's more, there will be ups and downs along the way, even with the willingness to accept your current situation. Most people think getting better is a straight and easy road, going from point A to point B, but that's just not realistic. Health is a journey along a winding road. With detours, speed bumps, stops, and panoramic views. Through this process, you're

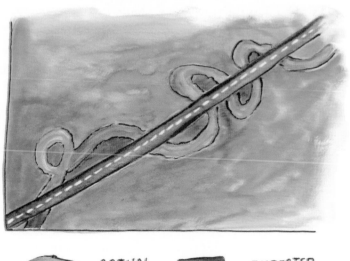

given a chance to grow, get out of your comfort zone, push your limits, and see your health and life through a different lens. It's an inner opportunity to learn more about yourself and take care of yourself so you can reach your highest potential in whatever life has to offer you.

You need to leave space for good days and bad. Just as there's enough room in the sky for a few thunderstorms, so too is there enough room in our mind for a few unpleasant thoughts and feelings.[116] Flare-ups, although distressing, are common and nothing to worry about. You're not getting worse, and you're not back at square one. Think of it as that resistance analogy I just shared with you. There's going to be some resistance during the process of change because you're challenging old habits and patterns. But here's the reality of it: there's the pain of staying the same and then there's the pain of change. Either road you take, discomfort and unpleasant feelings will surface. Naturally, there will be days where your body's going to throw a temper tantrum, and that's perfectly okay. Let it scream and shout, but don't cave in. It's kinda like that kid at the store you see screaming on the floor for their parent to buy them a toy. As uncomfortable and embarrassing as it is for the parent, they know not to cave because the minute they do, their little kiddo knows that all they have to do is put on this performance every time they want attention. Same goes for pain.

There are negative and positive reinforcement patterns of persistent pain that are helpful and some that are not so helpful or some that were once helpful but no longer serving you in the way that they once did. You might find yourself avoiding certain activities and experiences in life for fear that it will make things worse or cause more harm, but even that has been shown to be an ineffective strategy to cope with pain, one that only serves to ramp up fear and further avoidance even when the same strategies and behaviors fail to ease pain.[117] To put it another way, we keep doing the same ol' shit even when it's no longer beneficial and when the original purpose has long since passed. Imagine that your house is on fire. You run outside and grab what you think are buckets of water to put out the fire until your neighbor screams, "Hey, maybe you should put down the gasoline and try water!"

Oh, and remember all that talk about the brain? Don't forget that many things could be a trigger to set off your highly sophisticated threat-detection system. Take some time to think about what those triggers might be. Pay attention to how your body feels throughout the day and jot it down. You'll most likely find a pattern or theme. Being aware of your body and mental habits gives you the freedom to respond in ways that help you engage with the world (and your body) in a more meaningful way. Later on, you'll get a chance to create a flare-up plan so you'll be well equipped to handle them. Flare-ups, no problem. We'll have you covered!

ALL ABOUT CONTEXT

Let's say you're having the week from hell. You're behind on all your projects, the car's giving you trouble, you're eating like shit and sleep is nonexistent, you're fighting with your partner, oh and to top it all off, you just found out that you can't have those vacation days. Just an all-round craptastic week. Then you decide: *Screw it, I need a release. I'm going to masturbate.* Nothing wrong with that. But damn, there's a flare-up! Talk about a cock block. This time around it's unbearable, lasting longer than normal. For someone whose nervous system is already on high alert, it's no wonder your alarm bells are going off louder than normal. You've had a hellish week after all.

See how it's all about the context of the situation? Your week was shitty, so naturally psychophysiological reactions will follow. Reactions like increased tension, feeling more on edge, and experiencing amplified pain. This is completely normal. We all experience detours along the journey.

Now, let's say the opposite were true. Let's say you're having the best week of your life! You got that promotion, you went camping with your friends, you played soccer for the first time in years. And guess what. It wasn't so bad. No flare-ups. This time when you ejaculate, your pain's not nearly as high, almost nonexistent. Surprised? You shouldn't be. It's probably because of the situation. The week was great. You had some fun. As a result, your body released powerful neurochemicals to dampen danger messages. And voilà! You felt more at ease.

Every person responds differently to sensory stimuli depending on the context. You've probably experienced this yourself with the weather. You might feel chilly with certain temperatures while others feel warm. I've seen people wearing sandals and shorts in the dead of winter in Chicago. I actually know a guy who had a conversation with a friend for 30 minutes, barefoot in the snow. Examples like these should be proof enough to show that sensory stimulation is not the sole factor when it comes to the conscious experience of any sensation. It might not be a surprise to you, but this *includes* the sensation of pain.

The experience of pain also changes when you're persuaded either visually or verbally about what you *should* feel. Take for example this 2007 study by Moseley and Arntz[118] in which 33 study participants had a -20°C (-4°F, brrrr that's cold!) rod placed on the back of their hand. They were told that there would be a variety of probe temperatures even though only one temperature was used during the whole experiment. The researchers primed participants by planting verbal and visual persuasion about what to expect from the rod stimuli. They told people that the red light meant hot and the blue light meant cold, which naturally implies hot would be potentially more damaging and cold less damaging, given an implicit association of 'red is danger' and 'blue is safe'. There were also moments where participants could see the actual rod touch their hand with the associated light cue and instances where they were told to look away from the actual stimulus, but could still see the red or blue light cues. The authors found that people reported more pain when given the red-light cue prior to the rod touching their skin and when they had the opportunity to see the probe touch their skin in addition to the red-light cue. Keep in mind that the rod's temperature was always -20°C no matter which light cue was shown. The only thing that changed was what the participants *saw* and what they were *told* in relation to the stimulus. In this case, the rod's temperature didn't matter. The power of persuasion and the participants' preconceived meaning of red and blue is what influenced their sensory perception and threat detection. Again, all this to prove that sensory messages coming from your tissues alone are not sufficient to produce pain or trigger a sense of threat to your body or to you as a person.

So, next time your pain feels worse, take a step back to analyze your life in the recent weeks. What's been going on? Can you identify some possible triggers? The better you get at realizing what makes your pain tick, the better you'll be able to prepare and possibly prevent those flare-ups. Awareness is key. Karl Monahan, sports massage therapist and owner of The Pelvic Pain Clinic, has a great YouTube video on how to manage flare-ups. You can watch it here: https://youtu.be/ZmkepGYcjzc. The *Explain Pain Handbook Protectometer* is another great tool you can use to help you deepen your understanding of pain and discover those triggers. You can learn more about it at: http://www.protectometer.com/.

It's not just the outer context that matters; it's also the inner context that drives your experience of pain. I've had many people tell me that their pain suddenly got better (in some cases even disappeared) the moment they scheduled an appointment. Why is that? Pain motivates us to take action, and your brain was probably satisfied with your decision to seek out help from someone who understands your current predicament. Persistent pain not only challenges you physically, but it also threatens everything that brings meaning and purpose to your life. It can challenge your very existence as a human, and may prompt you to reevaluate your values and goals in life and contemplate deep philosophical questions like the meaning of life. The struggle is real.

Incessant pain can make anyone question the meaning and purpose of life, but what if pain was seen as a challenge instead of a threat? To quote psychiatrist and Holocaust survivor, Viktor Frankl: "Everything can be taken from a man but one thing: the last of the human freedoms – to choose one's attitude in any given set of circumstances, to choose one's own way."[119]

It's the ability to say yes to life and still find meaning to persevere and thrive. As if I haven't belabored the point enough, your outlook on your current situation influences your pain intensity and overall health. People who are able to find some good in a shitty situation generally experience positive physical health, better wellbeing, and less pain.[120] [121]

Now, I'm not saying that you can think happy thoughts and your pain will go away (if only it were that simple). Cultivating this mind of optimism is an internal job, and for some people this comes more naturally. For others, it takes some work to expose this potential. It also takes working with a team that can shine a light on your situation, exploring opportunities for positive experiences, guiding you to find your best self, and taking a stand for you when you want to give up. Finding meaning and purpose in life can be challenging for any human being, but it can be especially difficult during times of great distress, so it's important to wrap yourself up in resources that foster meaning-oriented care and a safe space for compassionate exploration. No matter how shitty a situation you find yourself in, there are always opportunities to thrive. Nature proves this to us all the time. Even in the harshest of climates, you'll always find tenacity, signs of life where you least expect it.

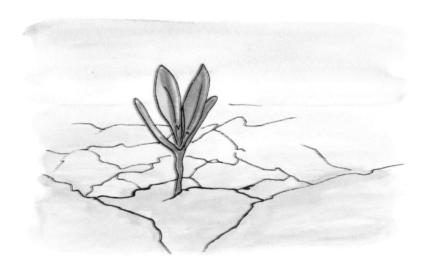

CHAPTER 5

ALL SYSTEMS GO

What do your gut, peeing, pooping and sex all have in common? When it comes to the body's systems... everything! They're interconnected processes that function together to keep you healthy and, ahem, *strong* in the erection department. The function and gusto of our bodily systems depend on our lifestyle choices to counterbalance environmental burden, stress, and the daily demands of being human. It's time to bridge the gap between your gut health, your penis and everything in between.

Did you ever feel butterflies in your stomach going out on a first date? Your brain and gut talk to each other. They go back and forth like a two-way highway. Brain-gut, gut-brain. In fact, the nervous system of the gut actually has its own special name – the enteric nervous system – to distinguish it from the brain and spinal cord. The gut-brain axis regulates the neuroendocrine (nervous and hormone system) and immune functions. So technically, we're talking about the brain, spinal cord, nervous system and gut all sharing the same phone plan.

What happens when they all share the same phone plan? If one goes over the minutes, the entire bill goes up, that's what. This is what happens to the body. If you're in distress, this will signal a cascade of events trickling from the brain to your gut and through the rest of your body, including the gut bacteria. And vice versa. Garbage in, garbage out. What you eat and how you live your life can alter your cellular health and create the same rippling effect up and down the chain.

WHAT'S ALL THIS ABOUT MY GUT?

The microorganisms living in your gut communicate with your central nervous system, which means your gut health can impact your mood, concentration, immune system, urinary tract, bowels and – you guessed it – pain.[122] [123]

The microbiome is not static. This ecosystem of microorganisms adapts and evolves with the environment, and as the host organism (you) changes and evolves. It's not uncommon for people to be on lots of medications (such as antibiotics), which disrupt the microorganisms that live in the gut and the urogenital tract. We all have 'good' and 'bad' bugs that live in harmony all over our body and are necessary for our health. When this balance gets disrupted, the body does a great job bringing it back into check, but sometimes it needs a little helping hand. The overall stress load on the body will determine whether your body's ecosystem is in harmony or not. So, things like your environment (like work and home life), your diet and exercise habits, smoking, medications, your sleep habits, your genetics, and any perceived threat to your body or you as a person (and with pelvic pain there's almost always a sense of this) all play a role in the health of your microbiome.

The ongoing fear, anxiety, and hopelessness that accompany persistent pelvic pain also alter this dynamic ecosystem balance via physiological stress response mechanisms. Stress, no matter what kind, activates nerves that alter the process of digestion, which can influence how much energy we absorb from nutrients, but also the time it takes to digest food. Lengthy digestion can put more stress and strain on the intestinal tract.[124]

Researchers aren't able to say confidently that altered gut or urinary microbiome is the *cause* for pelvic pain, but it may be another contributing factor to the perpetuation of ongoing pain and/or urinary issues (like overactive bladder, bladder pain syndrome, interstitial cystitis), again indicating that there's no single cause for woes down below.

Recall from Chapter 3 that there are complex pathways interconnected between the body, spinal cord, and your brain. All this information is being transmitted, adjusted, and analyzed depending on the overall balance of these systems. Any of these pathways can dampen or increase sensitivity of the overall system, leading to protection and activating the alarm bells. Remember that the main sensory messengers of your pelvic muscles are the pudendal nerve and its many branches originating from sacral spinal nerve roots S2-S4. These contain both sympathetic and parasympathetic neural fibers and connections (although even this understanding is not so cut and dry, and there is still much more to be learned when it comes to the autonomic nervous system), which communicate with all of your pelvic structures and the brain. So, there is much more at play in the way our privates work than we think.[125] [126] The pudendal nerve is motor and sensory, and involved with the autonomic nervous system, after all.[127]

As we have already covered, but is worth bearing in mind as we talk about the gut, one of the theories is that there is crosstalk between organs. One area may cross talk with another completely healthy region of the pelvis, contributing to referred pain via spinal neural and immune messengers and their neighboring branches. Information travels across several spinal segments, and along the way it picks up sensory information being relayed from other parts of your body coming in at the same time. Your gut is in close proximity to your pelvic area and shares many of the same neural pathways. So, if your gut or urinary health is not optimal, or there is inflammation in your colon, or if you're constipated, this can signal more protection from neighboring areas and vice versa. Lots of nosey neighbors checking in to make sure things are okay.

A 2016 study showed that gut microbiota could play an important role in CPPS. It showed that *prevotella* – a gram-negative bacteria mostly found in the gut, oral cavity, and vagina (if you have one) – was the lowest in men with CPPS. Interestingly enough, *prevotella* may play a role at reducing inflammation and is higher in people who eat a high fiber, high vegetable diet.[128] It's worth noting that there are many *prevotella* species some of which have even been shown to ramp up the immune response.[129] These unique bacterial ecosystems influence our health in different ways depending on where they take up residence and their respective ecological harmony. Of course, there are trillions of bacterial species that have yet to be discovered so we're just scratching the surface of the microbiota's influence on pelvic pain.

A healthy gut can decrease the inflammatory response in your body, enhance your mood, strengthen your immune system, and improve your sleep and pain.[130] Microorganisms change and adapt to environmental factors like stress, diet, and medication. The problem here is that most men will be on several courses of unnecessary antibiotic treatment, which has been shown to alter the gut microbiome. The aftermath of this can last weeks and even months after cessation of treatment.[131] [132] [133] All the while, symptoms persist. You've got no answers, making the distress rising, which doesn't help the gut issues. (See the cycle here?) Inflammatory-mediated pain mechanisms are influenced by what you put in your body and your overall lifestyle choices. You should know that the study of the microbiome is relatively new, and there's a lot that we don't know about the influence of these little buggers. We do know that there is an intimate interplay of these microorganisms on our health and wellbeing, so I'm excited to see what future research reveals about this connection.

Before I give you the detail on foods to eat and avoid, a word of recognition. I acknowledge that available food sources and affordability vary depending on where you live and what your current life circumstances are. This information is by no means intended to exclude or shame anyone. We work with the resources we have available.

Food is powerful medicine without side effects. What you put in your body will mirror how you feel. In fact, what you feed these microorganisms can change their composition and diversity in your gut in as little as a day![134] Processed sugar, fast food, fried foods, high saturated fats – to name a few – have been shown to be pro-inflammatory.[135] [136]And as you now know, inflammation increases the sensitivity of your pain and riles up your immune system. There's plenty of research to back up your parents' nagging about vitamins when you were a kid. We need basic nutrients to thrive like fatty acids (omega-3 and omega-6), vitamins, minerals (like magnesium, calcium and zinc), antioxidants, amino acids (building blocks of proteins), just to name a few. And to help us absorb and utilize these nutrients, we need the superpowers of bacteria!

Did you just get a brain freeze? Let me make this simple. **Eat. Real. Food.**

All of those nutrients that I just listed are found in fruits, veggies, dark leafy greens, fish, nuts, beans, olive oil... You get the gist. When it comes to taming your pain, you've got to consider tackling it from the inside out. And the next step is to consider what you're eating.

How would you describe your current diet? What does a healthy diet look like for you?

I hope I didn't just make you panic. I know how hard it is to make lifestyle changes, especially when it comes to food. I'm a foodie myself. So, let's take the pressure off a bit. If you're not ready to go cold turkey and stop eating pizza four nights a week, start adding some of these foods *into* your diet and slowly eliminate the junk. It's not going to be easy at first. Sugar's more addicting than cocaine. (Research shows 94% of cocaine-dependent rats made the switch to sugar given the choice, even when they had to work harder for it.)[137]

It's not just about what you're eating that matters either. It's also *how* you're eating as well. Eating on the go? Rushed? Distracted? How do you feel while you're eating? You've probably not considered the importance of thoroughly chewing your food to help your gut with the digestion process. Most of us forget that our stomach doesn't have teeth.

This is not to say that you can't indulge in your favorite foods from time to time. We all have our favorite comfort foods. Recognizing how you feel after eating certain foods will better guide you in making dietary decisions. And of course, seeking help from a licensed dietician or nutritionist for a more individualized approach to nutrition is recommended.

Regardless of the changes you decide to make in regards to your diet, know that change takes time. A healthy diet never goes out of style, so what do you have to lose by trying?

BLADDER IRRITANTS

Here's the skinny on bladder irritants. There's no single food or drink that is an absolute no-no. Everyone responds differently to what they eat and drink. So, can you drink Red Bull? Umm, it depends... on how much of this stuff you're drinking, on how you feel after drinking it and on other lifestyle factors. What creates a bladder annoyance for you might not be a bladder nuisance for the next dude. Remember, it's all about balance and being aware of your habits and how they serve you.

Once, I worked with a guy whose urge to pee all the time had come back. I asked if there had been any recent changes to his diet, stress, or sleep, and he responded that there hadn't. We were 30 minutes into the session when he told me about how he drank a few Red Bulls trying to pull an all-nighter driving home from a baseball game. Something that wasn't usual for him. Why am I not surprised the symptoms got worse? For one, he didn't get much sleep. And second, he drank a few Red Bulls (something that he hadn't drunk in a long time).

Red Bull, soda, coffee, iced tea, and any other caffeinated, sugary sweet beverages can potentially make your bladder go bonkers, especially if you've not had these items in a while. It's not that these things are inherently harmful; it's the dose and how your body responds to them that makes the difference. This can be especially important if there's an amplification of sensitivity of the bladder or bowel. Every person is different, but typically drinks that act like a diuretic (make you pee often) might exacerbate your symptoms.

Here are some other potential bladder and bowel irritants:
- Spicy foods
- Coffee
- Fizzy drinks
- Caffeine
- Alcohol
- Cigarettes

Again, these have been shown to aggravate bladder pain and urinary symptoms, but no direct causal link has been found.[138] And if you still don't believe me that processed sugar is kryptonite, a 2011 study in the *American Journal of Clinical Nutrition* showed that low to moderate sugar-sweetened beverage consumption promoted inflammation in healthy young men within just three weeks. Even at the lowest dose of 40g/day, changes were seen.[139] And they were being generous with that low dose. According to the American Heart Association, you should consume no more than about 25-37g sugar/day. To put it in perspective, one 12oz can of Coke has 39g of sugar in it! There goes your day's worth. So, the next time you grab a beverage, check out the ingredients and the nutritional label. You might be surprised at what you discover.

Alcohol is a touchy subject, but I'm gonna shine the light on it anyway. Although alcohol has been shown to have analgesic effects on pain, the risks (like excessive alcohol use and addiction) might outweigh the benefits in the long run.[140] Alcohol impacts your bladder function, but it can also be a doozy for your cardiovascular health, sexual function, immune defense mechanisms, microbiome, sleep, cognitive function, and your central nervous system.[141] [142] Not to mention all the sugar from alcohol has to metabolize somewhere. All of which can influence your pain sensitivity.

How much is too much? Well, that depends on you. Or more accurately, on your genes, your tolerance, your response, how you feel after drinking alcohol, and your allostatic load (cumulative burden on your bodily systems and mind). This not only applies to alcohol but also other changeable lifestyle factors that rev up the cumulative wear and tear on your body and your mind. Every body responds differently to alcohol. If this is a relevant discussion for you, you'll have to reflect and think hard about the influence of alcohol in your life. I'm not saying that you won't be able to enjoy a cocktail every now and then, I'm merely suggesting that you take into consideration the influence that alcohol might have on your current situation, your overall lifestyle, health and wellbeing.

Since we're on the topic of peeing, let's talk about poop. Everybody's favorite!

THE SCOOP ON POOP

If you're 'hulking it' to pop out that turd, we need to talk. Digestive issues can impact pelvic pain. For example, IBS (irritable bowel syndrome) has been associated with CPPS.[143] Altered gut microbiome and pooping habits can contribute to symptoms of abdominal pain, bloating, visceral pain, constipation, and diarrhea. Not to mention the excess distress placed on abdomo-pelvic structures. If it's difficult or painful to poop, it's only natural that your pelvic muscles are going to tense up and 'guard' every time you're dropping a deuce.

So, how do we address this issue? Two things: toileting posture and breath. In short, you want to sit like 'the Thinker' and breathe. How you sit on the throne affects the function of your pelvic floor muscles.

Rectum *damn near killed 'em*. Get it? Rec-tum as in 'wrecked him.' Okay, just trying to lighten the mood over here.

The rectum sits naturally in the pelvis with a 'bend in the hose' so to speak, getting help from your pelvic floor muscles to make sure you don't go around pooping yourself.

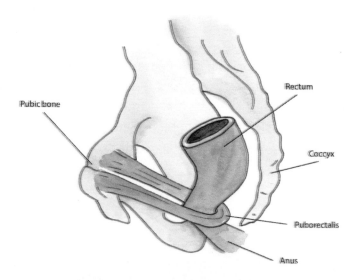

Puborectalis muscle wrapping around rectum

When you sit down on the toilet in an upright posture, these muscles semi-slacken, which makes it just slightly easier to poop without straining.[144]

Imagine what it would feel like to poop if the tube were straighter to allow for better outflow. The solution? A poop stoop. Ta-dah!

Before the luxury of toilets, people were known to squat to drop. Think of the last time you went camping, no Porta-Potty in sight. What did you do? Ass to grass, right?

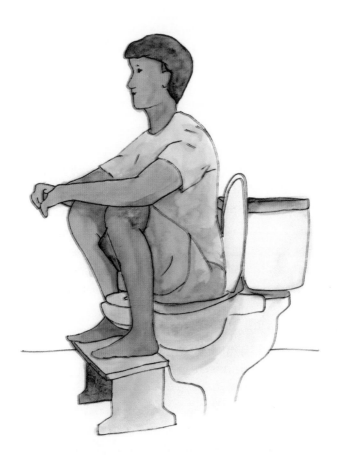

Step 1: Squat To Drop

Using a step stool under your feet will help bring the floor closer to you to mimic that optimal position, promoting a straighter rectum to make the flow flawless.

Rest your forearms on your knees keeping your back relaxed and knees apart. Like a person deep in thought.

Step 2: Breathe

Take a belly breath in. As you breathe out, gently tighten your abdominal muscles, if you need to push. If you can, avoid holding your breath while pushing down. This increases downward pressure on the pelvic diaphragm, which might cause the pelvic muscles to tighten reflexively instead of letting go. When this happens it's like trying to squeeze toothpaste out with the cap on. Eventually, prolonged straining and increased stress on the pelvic floor might result in hemorrhoids, painful bowel movements, bleeding, and/or an aggravation of your pain altogether.

Step 3: Give Yourself Time!

It's okay to give yourself time on the toilet (with number one and number two). Don't rush it. Rushing things might cause you to strain forcefully 'just to get it over with', or even feel 'not all the way done', which can also contribute to changes in bowel habits, bloating or frequent unnecessary trips to the bathroom.

On the flip side, you don't want to spend hours on the toilet straining, or sitting and staring at your phone. Excess pressure from sitting on the toilet 'too long', while mightily straining or pushing, might increase stress and strain of the tissues around the anus and rectum, potentially increasing pain, risk of hemorrhoids or, in rare cases, rectal prolapse, where the rectum starts to go down the path of least resistance. (Do yourself a favor and don't google this! Trust me on this one.)

How long is too long? Some literature reports more than 10 minutes being too long, but the reality is we really don't know what is too much time to spend on the toilet, as there are many other factors that can influence bowel health, some of which I have already touched upon like diet, lifestyle, stress, pooping habits, gut health, tissue genetics, even where you live in the world.[145][146] I don't necessarily believe that it's the *length* of time you sit on the toilet that's the trouble. It more likely has to do with excessive straining and pushing, and your overall health and fitness.

A biologically plausible reason (and a time saver) would be to suggest that if you don't have flow after five minutes or so, zip up and try again later. Another good indicator that you've sat too long is if your legs start going numb; at which point, it's probably best to get up and go. Risk factors for things like hemorrhoids haven't been adequately studied and further investigation is needed to make evidence-based claims for toilet habits. Until we have more information, keep things simple for yourself: get to know your body and your flow; there's no one way to poop.

MINDFUL POOPING

Do you ever bring your cell phone or electronic gadget into the bathroom with you? Come on, we're all guilty of it. And hands up who checks their email or uses this time to catch up on politics, social media and whatnot? Here's the thing, in a world full of distraction and stressors, it's easy for us to get sidetracked and lose ourselves in our devices.

Next time you bring your device to the bathroom for a number two, pay attention to what your body feels like. What do your shoulders and neck feel like? How's your breathing? Is it shallow or deep? Depending on what you're reading, playing or browsing, your body is most likely physically reacting to it, distracting you from the present moment and your intention to let go and let flow.

A body and mind under stress aren't going to get the 'this is a good time to poop' signal, remember? Ultimately, this can alter the process of digestion and elimination resulting in troublesome bowel habits.

Shelly Prosko, a dear friend and colleague of mine, came up with a clever acronym to help you get the most out of your toileting time. It's called AIRBAG. I encourage you to give it a try, especially if you've got trouble going number one or number two.

To paraphrase, this means:

Awareness: Do a quick scan of how your body and mind are feeling. No judgment or trying to change anything. Just observe and tap into that inner awareness.

Imagination: Bring to mind the image of your pelvic muscles as they span across from sitz bone to sitz bone, tailbone to pubic bone. Visualize the muscles, organs and the rest of the pelvic area doing their job, letting go and letting flow, feeling healthy and well.

Release: Soften the pelvic muscles and trust that your body knows exactly what to do.

Breathe: Tune into your natural breathing pattern, trying to not change it in any way. Allow the respiratory and pelvic diaphragms to dance to the tune of their own rhythm.

Allow: Allow yourself to let go (literally and figuratively) and explore what your body needs in the moment. Maybe you need to add a gentle push? Wiggle your butt on the seat? Lean back or lean forward? Allowing is giving yourself permission to feel and do what's right for your body, and not worry about how you *should* be pooping.

Gratitude: If you really think about it, it's pretty damn amazing how your body is able to perform such complex processes every day of your life without you having to think twice about it. Take a second to appreciate this process and all that your body continues to do for you moment by moment.

For the full guided version of Shelly's 'toilet meditation', visit her original blog post here: www.physioyoga.ca/the-6-stages-of-toilet-meditation

CATCH THOSE ZZZZS

Let's take a brief sleep audit.[147]

Do you get less than 5-6 hours of sleep per night?

Do you feel tired when you wake up in the morning even after getting 7-8 hours of sleep?

Do you experience difficulty falling asleep at night? Or difficulty returning back to sleep when you wake up in the middle of the night?

Is your pain impacting your sleep? If so, how?

Do you snore loudly or frequently?

Do you have a strong urge to move your legs continually while trying to sleep?

Do you get lots of screen time? If so, do you use a blue light filter?

If you answered 'yes' to more than a couple of the questions above, we need to have a chat about your sleep. And we definitely need to take a look at your sleep hygiene or bedtime routine.

It doesn't matter if you're a night owl or an early bird, as long as you're getting restful sleep. Your body needs this time to repair and rejuvenate to prepare you for the challenges of the next day. Difficulty sleeping and persistent pain go together like peanut butter and jelly.

Your sleep quality can predict the level of pain you have the following day. Poor sleep increases sensitivity and disability.[148] Stress, pain, anxiety, worry, fear and so on amp up neuroendocrine responses in the body, which tend to impact sleep (and digestion). Why? The short version goes like this (though there are a lot more hormones in play, and it does get a lot more complicated). For the sake of what we're taking about here, the important part to know is that cortisol, the stress hormone, runs on a circadian rhythm. Typically, it peaks first thing in the morning, gradually drops throughout the course of the day and reaches the lowest point at night. That means the protective mechanism used in your fight or flight mode – cortisol – is supposed to be lower at night. However, if it's on overdrive or disrupted, over time, cortisol doesn't function to reduce inflammation, and it will make your symptoms seem like they're much worse, especially during times of fluctuation. For example, during the day, you're distracted, flying high on adrenaline. Come bedtime, though, your ammunition runs low, so it's easier for your brain to pay attention to your body, including the aches and pains.

Sleep is important because without it your body doesn't rest and repair, continuously perpetuating the physiological stress response cycle and making your nervous system more sensitive to daily demands. It's also important for immune function, tissue healing, pain modulation, cardiovascular health, cognitive function, learning and memory.[149] While you sleep you also have microglial cells, specialized immune cells in the CNS, that do a little neural pruning, a bit like pulling out weeds in your brain's garden. This 'clean-up' creates space for new learning, making neural connections more streamlined and efficient. This is particularly important as you're trying to plant seeds of new neuronal pathways to replace those connections associated with your pain experience.[150]

GETTING THE BEST OUT OF YOUR SLEEP

It's not only the kiddos that need a bedtime routine. Adults need them too. If you're having a hard time shutting off your brain at night, try to build a better bedtime ritual. Create a more suitable environment to make sure you're getting those zzzs. Too much artificial light can throw off your sleep-wake patterns. This includes your computer, phone, and any other screens. So, if you're up all night glued to a screen, you might want to start thinking of some new bedtime habits.

Start by tapping into your current bedtime routine. What does bedtime look like for you? How does your body feel? What are you doing? Do you look forward to sleeping or do you dread it?

According to Dr. Rubin Naiman, a clinical psychologist specializing in integrative sleep and dream medicine, "Sleep is an experience." If you're tossing and turning, getting frustrated that you can't fall asleep, this may be a part of the problem. Like accepting your pelvic pain, you need to start accepting your sleeplessness. The anxiety and effort in paying attention to all the things in your life that are 'not going so well' only creates more tension, adrenaline, and anxiety around the very thing you're fighting so hard against. Dr. Naiman suggests, "Sleep will naturally and gradually begin to seep through when we let go of effort. Relinquishing sleep effort is about letting go of our waking self – our sense of who we believe we are. It's about willingly losing the battle for control of sleep by realizing that falling asleep cannot be controlled. Sleep is, in essence, a free ride for all those who are simply willing to be passengers."[151] Hmmm, sounds like you could relate this to your pain experience as well.

I'm going to rattle off some tips for better sleep, but remember, you're unique and should customize a routine for your lifestyle.[152] There's no one-size-fits-all.

- ➤ Go to sleep and wake up at the same time every day. This trains your biological clock.
- ➤ Switch off that blue light! Shut down your TV, phone, tablet, or whatever you use for one to two hours before bed.
- ➤ If you need a nap, keep it to 20 minutes or less.
- ➤ Avoid drinking alcohol in the evening. This will save you on trips to the bathroom in the middle of the night.
- ➤ If letting go of technology is too hard, try using a blue light filter. You can get one called F.lux at: justgetflux.com

- ➤ No caffeine, sugary drinks or snacks before bedtime.
- ➤ Wind down. Maybe you like journaling? If journaling isn't for you, try meditation. I'm not all against the use of technology. Try listening to a podcast called *Sleep with Me* that you can find at: sleepwithmepodcast.com
- ➤ Take a bath.
- ➤ Use your bed for sleep and sexual activity only. No snacking, reading or watching TV.
- ➤ Keep your bedroom dark and cool.
- ➤ Don't pump iron right before bed. High impact, adrenaline-pumping exercise energizes your body. Not a good idea if you're having trouble falling asleep. But make sure you are exercising, preferably in the morning.
- ➤ If you're going to watch TV, try watching something that's relaxing, fun, and lighthearted. Watching a nail-biter right before bed will flick on your fight or flight response mechanism, which isn't helpful when trying to get to sleep.
- ➤ Don't work so hard in the evening. Just like your body, your mind needs a break too.
- ➤ Breathe yourself to sleep. Focused belly breathing helps lower your heart rate, decreases tension in muscles, lowers your blood pressure, and stimulates the rest-and-digest nervous system.
- ➤ Go play outside! The more natural sunlight you get, the better your sleep cycle.

And if pain isn't enough to convince you to clean up your sleeping habits, maybe your boner will. Yup, quality sleep also means quality erections.[153] [154]

IT'S 'GETTING HARD'

All this talk about pelvic pain and poop is getting hard, I know, maybe even overwhelming. But that's not what I'm getting at here. Next up, I'm talking about boners. And exercising your right to pleasure yourself.

Despite what you think you know, many guys don't actually have the full lowdown on how this body part operates. But if you're interested in achieving a pain-free erection – and I think you are! – it's important to understand how it requires a team approach between your mind, musculoskeletal system (yup, pelvic muscles), endocrine system, nervous system and vascular system. Of course, when pain is in the bedroom, this can dampen any party in your pants. Completely normal, given the circumstances. Understanding how your penis functions will help you troubleshoot your erections even in the face of pain.

So, here's a brief tutorial on how your penis works. When you stimulate your genitals, the sensory nerves of your penis (pudendal nerve and its branches) fire, sending messages to specific areas of your spinal cord. These messages then activate nerves that go to your pelvic muscles, which jump-start the bulbospongiosus and ischiocavernosus muscles to contract. In addition, achieving and maintaining an erection depends on the neural and chemical interplay between the sympathetic and parasympathetic nervous systems. The sympathetic nervous system is the default mode when your penis is not in use. This constant sympathetic neural flow keeps norepinephrine, along with other chemicals, circulating within the erectile tissue to keep your boner at bay until you're ready to play. For an erection to occur, the parasympathetic nervous system revs up and takes over, signaling the release of a powerful molecule called nitric oxide (NO) within the erectile tissue. This relaxes the arteries in your penis to allow increased blood flow into the penis. As the erectile tissue expands, it compresses the veins in the penis to prevent blood flow from sneaking out. The pelvic muscles help with your erection by squeezing around the base of the penis allowing you to manipulate movement, blood flow and firmness of your penis. They also rhythmically squeeze and release during ejaculation to expel semen.[155][156] Sounds simple, right? If only it were.

Getting an erection isn't just about genital touch and spinal reflexes. You can also get an erection thinking, seeing, hearing, or smelling any stimulus that is erotic (to you) or triggers arousal. That being said, everyone is unique, and what turns you on might be a turn off for someone else. The most important organ involved for arousal and erection is the one that sits between your ears. Your brain! There are areas of the brain that regulate sexual arousal via neural, hormonal, and chemical processes. The brain also has the power to modulate the activity levels of the sympathetic and parasympathetic nervous systems, communicating with the nerves all the way down to your genitals. Signals from the brain can also make the nerve endings in your genitals extra sensitive, which is great for pleasure but not so fun with pain in the bedroom.

A problem anywhere on the path from the brain, spinal cord or nerves to the penis can put a damper on the fun 'down there.' And all it takes is one time when things don't work well to build worry in your mind about the next time, and the next, and the next, which is why it can be doubly worrisome with pelvic pain.

Your penis doesn't know the difference between a bear chasing you or a 'what if it happens next time?' worry. Both situations use the same physiological process to disrupt arousal, erections, and fun: igniting the sympathetic nervous system, that fight or flight response.

Neurohormonal chemicals such as norepinephrine and adrenaline can pour cold water on any party in your pants. These chemicals reduce the effects of nitric oxide to shunt blood away from your penis to greater areas of need like your heart, big muscle groups, and brain. You might not be running away from a bear, but daily chronic stressors can have a similar impact, especially if you're worried or anxious about what's going on *down under*, such as with pelvic pain.

Just because you couldn't 'lift off' one time doesn't mean you're going to have a heart attack or not be able to perform the next time. Performance worry is common and can happen to anyone. You're not 'broken.' There's a lot to be said about the context of any given situation that you're in. Your response and outlook on what's happening will change the outcome. Sound familiar?

HOW ABOUT HORMONES?

And let's not forget about the influence of the hormone system on your erections. Testosterone and other hormones influence cognitive function, mood, and sexual and musculoskeletal health. It's common for testosterone levels to change with age and your lifestyle. It's been re-ported that testosterone levels may decrease 1-2% per year from your individual baseline (depending on if and when you get tested and how your levels change over time).[157] This rate of change also depends on en-vironmental and lifestyle factors like diet, exercise, stress, and sleep.[158]

But how low is too low? There's actually no 'normal' value better than your own baseline for comparing testosterone levels. Most lab tests use wide reference ranges, including for age, which means they are not indi-vidually specific. Plus, all labs represent a snapshot in time as biological processes change and can be altered in any given moment, so it's wise to repeat testing a few times to have a more reliable measure. According to the American Urological Association (AUA), 300 ng/dl is the recom-mended cut-off score for low T. Of course, this is taken into consider-ation with other laboratory testing in addition to your accompanying signs or symptoms that may be indicative of too low testosterone. [159]

Sometimes your number can look normal on blood tests, but tes-tosterone may still not be working properly in your body, which would necessitate more investigation. Your levels might not compare to the reference range, but that's okay as long as you're feeling great and your love muscle is functioning strong.

Testosterone levels shouldn't be taken at face value or used to diag-nose anything just on their own. As I said, there are many other hor-monal influences at play here. Instead, consider them in conjunction with your reported symptoms and the overall picture.

Is there a connection between low T and pelvic pain in men? I hit the books, researching near and far for the answer. And you know what I came up with? Nothing. Okay, I didn't come up entirely empty-hand-ed, but the research about this topic is slim to none. I didn't call it quits there. I kept digging and put together some of my own thoughts based on the research.

When you suddenly get pain 'down there,' a ripple of events usually happens. You go see an MD, who most likely gives you some antibiot-ics and then sends you on your merry way. A month or so goes by and you feel a little better with the meds, but the pain comes back. So, you go back to the doctor, and they give you another round of antibiotics…

And then another... And another. By now, it's probably been a good seven or eight months, maybe even a year dealing with this nightmare. You're frustrated, pissed, and feeling hopeless. You've seen too many doctors and gotten no answers. You might've been told you're just going to have to live with this for the rest of your life – the ultimate death sentence that sends you over the edge. (No joke, some clinicians are still saying things like this to guys in pain. It's not their fault. They only know so much and get intimidated by conditions like persistent pelvic pain because they just don't know how to help you. Don't get me wrong. They all have good intentions, but they might've just exhausted all the tools in their toolbox.)

Hearing this doesn't mean you should crawl into a dark hole and sulk. It means that there are other wellness professionals with other perspectives who might help you get the results you want. There's hope. Unfortunately, because you're only human, you start doubting your ability to get over this, and the worry, anxiety and distressing thoughts looping around and around in your head start controlling your life. Although quite normal to experience for any human, if allowed to run the show for long, these thoughts can have negative impacts on your overall health and wellbeing. It's no wonder that over half of men with persistent pelvic pain have depression and – drumroll please – erection problems.

Now, remembering that stress and anxiety impact your pain, sleep, hormone, immune and nervous systems, here's what happens next. Stress (including many complex physiological pathways) sets off the fight or flight response mechanisms of the body. Doing this releases protective chemical hormones like cortisol, adrenaline, norepinephrine. So far, so normal. We've gotten to grips with this in previous chapters.

Over time, though, the release of these protective chemicals impacts the complex pathways that modulate the production and synthesis of your hormones. Testosterone levels aren't just altered by stress. They can fluctuate based on your sleep patterns, diet, inflammation in the body, pain, gut microbiome, exercise habits, etc.

So, can low testosterone be the major contributing factor for your symptoms? Most likely not. Very few studies have shown any relationship. One study did suggest that low T symptoms and 'prostatitis-like' symptoms may have a connection, but the research was not strong enough to support any claim, admitting, "We believe that T can affect CP/CPPS but only to a limited extent because the cause of CP/CPPS is multifactorial."[160]

Bottom line: There are many other systems in play that feed off of each other, so we can't point the finger solely at low T for the cause of pelvic pain.

TO MASTURBATE OR NOT?

Again, my answer here is it depends. During ejaculation, your pelvic floor muscles squeeze and release several times to pump semen out of your penis. It's a workout for your pelvic floor muscles, but this is completely natural and normal, something you probably never even paid attention to until now. It's when this process becomes painful (during or afterwards) that there's an issue. What was once an experience of pleasure is now fraught with danger. Talk about mixed messages.

Pelvic muscles and surrounding tissues are built to tolerate and withstand such demands, but when the sensitivity dial is turned up loud, something so natural can be enough to trigger the alarm bells, especially at a time when you least expect it. The more these associations are made, the more you anticipate it to happen, further perpetuating fear and worry about the state of your affairs… in bed.

So, it's unsurprising that a common question is: should I stop masturbating or having sex? This decision is entirely up to you. Masturbation is not a *cause* for pelvic pain. And how much is 'too much' is subjective. There's little to no quality research on whether or not ejaculation makes symptoms of CPPS better or worse.

Despite the lack of evidence, I'm gonna be bold here and say that you don't need to masturbate to get better or vice versa. Depending on your spiritual, religious, cultural or personal beliefs and values, this might not even be an option and that's perfectly okay! Something else to consider here is masturbation techniques. Sometimes tissue trauma may result from excessive, aggressive, masturbation habits and other sexual behavior activities. Again, this will vary per individual and how much is 'aggressive' or 'excessive' is subjective.

Bottom line: Your own experience should guide you to decide what a healthy amount of sexual activity is for you.

This, however, can be tricky when there's a lot of fear around getting a flare-up post-ejaculation or even with an erection. That being said, you could explore dialing back from your usual sexual activity routine or frequency to see how you feel. Not forever, just temporarily. It's like with any other part of your body that's cranky. You work to calm things down and build things back up gradually. The same concept applies when you flex your sex muscles.

If something is painful, you won't desire it, including sex and intimacy. This means desire, arousal, and sexual function will be impacted. So, while you're working to calm things down, so you don't miss out on opportunities for pleasure, see if you can find other meaningful ways to pleasure-hunt to enrich your connection with yourself and/or your partner. This may push your comfort zone by challenging your current definition of sex and intimacy. These terms are concepts that don't have boundaries or rules, but mainstream culture may have you thinking otherwise. Consider what it would be like to reframe your sexual issues from problems to opportunities to find other ways to reconnect with yourself and your cock. Sex doesn't have to involve erections, penetration, or peak performance. You can experience pleasure without the firework show at the end.

Here's what I mean by that…

How has your sexual identity been affected by pelvic pain?

How else could you show your penis love without shame, blame or guilt?

What does sex mean to you?

What can you do to make sex meaningful despite pain?

What areas of your body feel safe to explore?

What would it take to trust in your body (ahem, your penis) again?

How would it feel to leave the pressure to perform out of it?

All these questions are geared towards bringing awareness back into your body, to re-establish a sense of safety, to reawaken your whole self as a sexual being and not just your penis. Sometimes, the 'rules' we set for ourselves around the concept of sex can limit us. Flexibility to embrace variability and vulnerability is important, so that when something does change (and it always will, because sexual pleasure and function are fluid and ever-changing based on context), we won't be so thrown off guard, upset or attached to things being a certain way.

Phew! That's been some learning curve in the last few chapters. Everything from poop to sleep, hormones to masturbation. Now that you've got a better understanding of the way your mind and body operate, it's time to put all of this into practice.

CHAPTER 6

THE NUTS AND BOLTS OF TREATING PELVIC PAIN

In this section of the book, I guide you through specific, practical self-help strategies to help ease your pelvic pain and plant some peace in your mind. I want to preface this by saying these suggestions aren't the be-all-and-end-all solution to your problems. No miracle cure. Every person responds differently to the various things they try. I encourage you to take this information and play with it. Explore, be curious, and most importantly listen to the wisdom of your body.

If you want to tweak some of the ideas below, go for it! In fact, I want you to. These are just suggestions, not rules. The best approach is the one that you individualize, make your own, and actually want to do. Remember, the purpose is for you to discover the inner expert in yourself so that you have the confidence and gumption to move forward with life even in the face of pain, worry, and fear. So, here's to choosing your own adventure!

MANAGING EXPECTATIONS

There's a positive feedback loop between your expectations and pain. The more you expect something to hurt, the greater your brain will respond to it; the greater your brain responds, the more it will hurt.[161]

In the Jepma et al work from 2018, the authors investigate the relationship between expectations and pain. As the saying goes: once bitten, twice shy. The expectation of pain intensity will change what

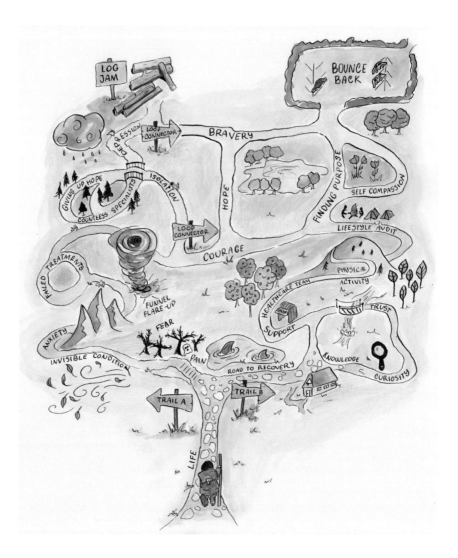

you feel and how the brain processes 'pain' even when what you expect doesn't occur, and regardless of whether the stimulus was actually noxious or not.[162]

Pessimistic expectations stick like Velcro and make it really hard to detach from negatively anticipated outcomes. All it takes is one bad experience. When it's with your genitals, this gets extra attention and extra sticky, a completely normal response. Although we might not be able to get rid of these protective mechanisms, we can change our relationship with them (our response). It takes practice and gathering evidence in defense of feeling good. Making the good more explicit and noticeable is important for shifting neurological patterns and learned behavior. We need to make the 'good' more noticeable.

Scientists have discovered that negative and positive expectations influence pain perception via complex neurophysiological pathways.[163] Expectations are persuaded by all your five senses, your previous experiences, what you've been told, what you've read, and what you've observed in others experiencing a similar situation. Negative persuasion has been shown to make harmless sensory stimulation rather painful and perceived just as strongly as if it were an actual noxious stimulus. On the flip side, positive expectations and persuasion have the power to detangle pain neurotags.[164] [165] [166] [167]

Otherwise put, success with new treatment may reduce as negative expectations and unpleasant experiences increase. Emotional and cognitive factors (our beliefs) also influence our expectations around a particular outcome.[168] All this to say that the language and words we choose and hear around the context of pain have the ability to help or hurt. Changing how we relate to pain has the ability to unlock some pretty powerful neurochemicals in our brain to help reduce pain.[169] Check out this video by Michael Stevens to experience the power of persuasion and the influence that anticipation and expectations have on touch and pain: https://youtu.be/OUdXMoY6fLY

Here's an idea to help make the positive (or less bad) more noticeable. Make yourself a 'win' jar to add to and reflect on positive experiences often. There is no win too small. Anything is worthy of celebrating.

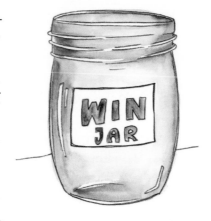

Speaking of expectations, this isn't easy for me to bring up, but it's important to be transparent here and remember that there will be crappy days, okay days, great days, good days. All of those are valid. There's a certain level of uncertainty we need to embrace as you navigate this journey. Although this is the reality of it, the approach doesn't have to suck. Instead of worrying about the what-ifs, let's make space in your mind for all the experiences that are yet to come. Making space means that you're willing to move towards pain rather than away. Instead of avoiding or enduring the inevitable, you become curious and take each moment that arises as a brand new moment, because that's exactly what it is. Every second that ticks is a brand new second to experience life. You'll never get it back. How you choose to experience that second is up to you.

So, before applying the strategies I'm about to share with you, ask yourself this question: am I ready to drop the struggle, the endless search for a cause, for cures, for the fix? I ask because sometimes the unrelenting and insatiable chase for cures and causes may be the thing that stops you from getting on with your life. It's like riding a rollercoaster, over and over and over again. Eventually the fun is over, making you more nauseous and sick than when you first got on. Lots of time, energy, and money is invested into riding the rollercoaster without the thrill or the fun.

I say this as if it were easy. It's not. It takes balls, literally. But in order to stop the nausea (and hopefully you're not vomiting), you need to step off the rollercoaster. Sometimes the simplest thing to do is the most counterintuitive. It's human nature to want to problem-solve, do, fix, rinse and repeat, but there comes a time when being is enough. Just being. Nothing else. Difficult situations will always be part of the human predicament, but they don't have to be problems. Buddhist monk Geshe Kelsang Gyatso once said, "If we were to respond to difficult situations with a positive and peaceful mind, they would not be problems for us; indeed, we may even come to regard them as challenges or opportunities for growth and development."[170]

Dropping the struggle doesn't mean you're throwing in the towel. Being at peace with what is presently happening in your life allows you to find a solution from a place of balance and with that comes peace, inner freedom and resilience. It's an understanding that outer problems are endless. If we really think about it, we can't control external circumstances no matter how hard we line up our ducks in a row. The only thing that we have control over is how we respond and how we react to any given situation. After all, what has anger and impatience ever solved? Again, this is simple, not easy.

It'll take practice and an understanding that change should be approached as a path not a destination. We're not born with this way of thinking, but consider this... The points of the compass – north, south, east and west – are directions not destinations. Viewing your health journey like this, as a path not a destination, may take some of the pressure off.

In addition, I encourage you to reflect on the strategies you've been using so far to see how they've been serving you on this journey. Have these strategies helped you in the long run, really? Do you believe you have the answer within yourself to feel and be well? Ultimately, you have the magic that you've been searching for all this time. You just need a little nudge to tap into this potential. Famous Italian sculptor Michelangelo envisioned the statue of David in a lump of rock. He saw the potential in what others considered to be worthless. I'm asking you to do the same for yourself moving forward.

TURN DOWN THE NEURAL NOISE

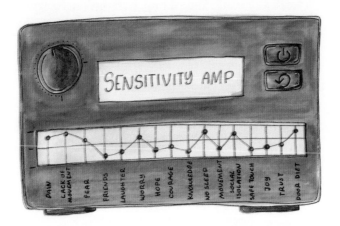

Guess what? You've already begun the process of turning down the sensitivity dial by equipping yourself with some pretty powerful knowledge just by reading this book so far. Pain scientists Dr. David Butler and Prof.

Lorimer Moseley say, "Knowledge is the greatest pain liberator of all!"[171] Understanding why you hurt makes the situation less scary. For one, now you know that you're not causing yourself more harm or damage when you venture to do the things you love despite feeling pain. Sure, it's uncomfortable, but knowing that the pain you're experiencing is a sensitive nervous system opens up a whole world of possibilities and options to reduce the neural noise. This understanding might even encourage you to dabble in activities that you thought would never be possible again.

There are many other ways to recalibrate the nervous system, like exploring with movement, safe touch, and the psychological aspects of health and wellbeing.

When you absorb yourself in activities you love, surround yourself with positive people, have a thigh-slapping laugh, use language that is uplifting, exercise, encounter positive, caring and empathetic health professionals, or get a dose of the 'hug drug,' you tap into your brain's own drugstore. Your brain has the capabilities of producing and releasing into your bloodstream some of the world's most powerful painkillers: endorphins like opioids, dopamine, oxytocin, morphine, serotonin and adrenaline just to name a few. They work better than any synthetic drug money can buy! When the flood gates open, these potent neurochemicals work their magic to dampen danger messages coming in from the body.[172] [173] [174] Don't believe me? Just ask American professional golfer Tiger Woods how he won the 2008 US Open tournament hobbling around with two stress fractures in his leg and a bum knee.[175] To learn more about the drug cabinet in your brain, check out this video: https://youtu.be/Gd2NaGZa7M4

FULL TO OVERFLOWING

First things first, let's find out what has been overflowing your cup. Pain is a balance of everything that's swirling around in your cup. It's also dependent on your cup's capacity for what it's holding. Depending on what's going on in your life, this cup may be slowly teetering on the verge of spilling, like when you get a latte that's filled up to the brim and the only way you're going to get it to your seat without spilling is to take a sip right off the top, then pray you don't slosh it all over the floor as you start walking. Or it might be half-full but with a flame underneath cranked up all the way. However you look at it, it's either a small, steady spillage over time or a roaring boiling overflow. Both need your attention! It's usually the resistance to 'roll with the punches' that trips people up.

Once you can recognize the factors that are influencing your health and wellbeing, you can then make a decision to do something or nothing about it. It's your choice.

Go ahead and grab a sheet of paper or draw this up on your tablet. If you're artsy, feel free to literally draw a cup leaving enough room inside to jot down the things in your life that are causing it to overflow. If you're like me and can barely draw a stick figure, just make a list. Don't overthink it. Take a few minutes to reflect on your whole life in the present moment. To do this, it might be helpful to take the perspective of an observer, as if you were watching a scene from your own life's movie. Now write down all the things in your life that are filling up your cup, making a huge mess on the floor and in your life.

Identifying underlying triggers that mediate and perpetuate protective responses (pain, anxiety, fear, distressing thoughts, physical stressors,

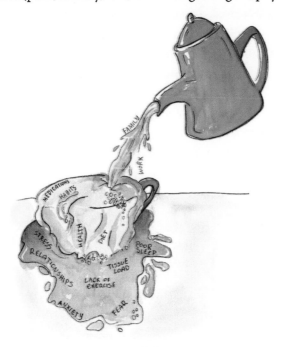

inflammation, etc.) will allow you to begin to recognize and adapt to these triggers to create safety for your nervous system. Whenever there is more conceivable evidence of danger than safety, the brain will decide to protect you.[176]

It's also beneficial to look for triggers that are positive and pain-reducing. To help you identify this, think about whether there are ever times in your day when you have less pain or don't notice it at all. This answer will guide you to do activities that will build up safety and calm your nervous system.

After you've jotted down your thoughts, contemplate each one of them individually and the influence they have on your life. What can you do to make more space in your cup, or what can you do to stop filling the cup? Even the slightest change can make space to prevent spillage. Sometimes there's lots we can do to change our circumstances, other times, not so much and that's okay. Our ability to adapt to any given situation builds physical and mental resilience.

It's not always easy reflecting on your own life in this way because there might be some serious issues to deal with. As the question goes: how do you eat an elephant? One bite at a time. You don't have to tackle everything at once. Just the fact that you took the time to put things down on paper and get them out of your head is therapeutic! Moving forward, admit to what you are willing to entertain as far as change goes and start there. If you're still having trouble figuring out where to start, ask yourself these questions:

How might someone else approach this [situation]?
What would you say to a friend who was going through this [situation]?

The answers to these questions aren't easy either, but they're here to help you reflect on your current situation through a different lens, a lens of compassionate inquiry.

DITCHING THE 'IN PAIN' IMAGE OF YOURSELF

Life's struggles might sometimes leave us feeling defeated and lost. The person who you once related to before pain might not be the same person who's reading this book right now. You might also be grieving the loss of your identity, maybe even friendships or your job. This detour in life can be quite devastating, no doubt.

It's oh-so easy to gravitate towards a negative mind when you're in pain. It's a human thing. Whenever you find your mind springing back to doom and gloom or thinking unhelpful thoughts and beliefs, that's because it's been practiced for a long time, eventually getting easier for your mind to move in that direction. Familiarity is what keeps pain set as your default mode, but it doesn't have to be this way. Just as quickly as you can change direction with one small pivot step, you can change how you relate to pain and move in a direction of greater peace and wellbeing.

Now, I don't know you personally, but I can definitely tell that pain is *not* the true, authentic version of you. You don't go around introducing yourself like this:

"Hi, I'm pelvic pain, nice to meet you."

Pain, just like everything else, is a familiar habit. And like all habits, it can be changed. When you think of yourself as a fixed, permanent self, it leaves little possibility for change. Naturally, then, you'll feel stuck. When you start to shift your perspective about pain and your current situation, you'll begin to feel less attached to the person in pain. As a result, pain will loosen its grip.

Try not to relate to that painful version of yourself no matter how many times it rears its ugly head. Instead, relate to the best version of yourself. When it does pop up – which it will – give thanks to your pain, because it's just another reminder of who you're not. Changing the version(s) that you normally identify with will be helpful in changing the relationship you have with pain and perhaps the diagnoses you received along the way, which may or may not have been helpful for you. The pain might still be there, but it doesn't have to be jumping all over your lap fighting for the TV remote when you're trying to relax. Instead, you're making room for pain to work with it in a meaningful way.

There are many unhelpful versions of self that we wear on a moment-to-moment basis, so why not clean out the closet and put on something new, fresh and more uplifting?

Roll up your sleeves. We've got some work to do!

When I say work, we'll be working in instead of the traditional working out. Doing this will help you recognize what's important to you in life and what will give you the space to engage with life in a meaningful and purposeful way. It's a way to create your own compass, because without direction, you would be lost (probably a bit like you're feeling right now).

There are many ways to go about this. One of my favorite ways is to create a vision board, more like a vision for yourself. This can be done the old-fashioned way with poster board, magazines, glue stick, markers, and any other arts and crafts you fancy. Or you can create a virtual board. Or you can journal your reflections. Or you can mind map. Any combination of these would work, and if you've done something else in the past that you really enjoyed as part of this reflection process, go for it!

Here are a few questions to ponder as you reflect on your vision:

How hopeful are you that things can get better?

What would 'better' look like for you?

How will you know when you get there?

How do you want to feel in your body?

How do you want to live your life?

What would you love to do?

How would you like to engage with the world?

Who or what inspires you?

How would your life change if pain were not an issue?

As you reflect on each question, notice how your body feels as you imagine, touch, see images and read words that represent your vision, that represent *you*. What does it feel like to have a sense of direction, a path to follow driven by your own internal compass?

One thing to note is that this vision is not fixed. Just as you're constantly evolving and changing, so will your vision. If you were to look at some old photographs, you would see that the person who you were back then is not the same person now. Your likes, dislikes, out-fits, hairstyle, choice of music, how you spend your weekends, all of these change as you evolve over time. Just more proof that your life, de-spite being in pain right now, is changing and will continue to change. Something to keep in mind!

Here's an example of a vision board done by one of my patients us-ing a word cloud. He uses this to remind himself of his path whenever the unexpected weather takes his boat off-course.

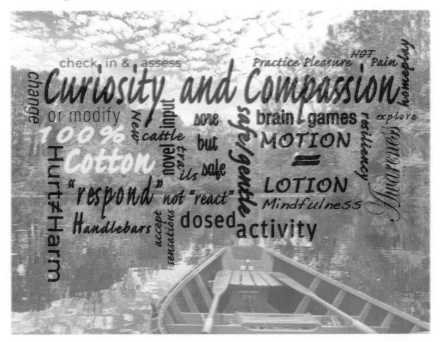

However you choose to reflect on your vision, it's helpful to keep it handy to remind you to stay on course, especially when the journey gets turbulent.

BREATHE IN THE GOOD SHIT, BREATHE OUT THE BULLSHIT

Breathing is an essential part of life that most of us take for granted. As I mentioned already in earlier sections of the book, focused dia-phragmatic breathing, AKA belly breathing, can be a game-changer.

I've seen it benefit many people in pain, and I'm confident it can do the same for you, too.

Typically, with pain, stress, anxiety, or excitement, your breathing patterns change. It might be shallower, faster, more rigid, or more tense in your chest or belly. Breathing pattern changes are common in the face of unexpected and acute pain. In fact, it's almost an involuntary reflex, which is a naturally driven process. Increases in respiratory rate (as with hyperventilation) during times of acute pain or distress are a respiratory stress response, another form of protection, just in case you need to fight or flee. This is functional and applicable for acute situations, but in chronic pain, we're not so sure how it influences breathing nor whether these same mechanisms are as beneficial in this context. Even the anticipation of pain can cause changes in your breathing pattern.

There are some biologically plausible theories that explain the mechanisms behind how slow and controlled breathing might decrease pain like via the cardiovascular system (heart rate and blood pressure), autonomic nervous system, central nervous system, and via behavioral factors like distraction, expectations and attention shift.[177] Most likely, it's a combination of all these things and more. Overall, the consensus seems to be: although there is no single 'right' way to breathe, slow, deep breathing does influence our physiology and can be a useful tool to modulate pain.

Here's a fun little activity you can do right now to see firsthand how breathing influences your heart rate. Find your pulse by placing two fingers on your wrist just below the meaty part at the base of your thumb.

Now, take a moment to pay attention to the natural rhythm of your pulse. While doing this, take a deep breath in and just linger a few counts at the end of your inhale. Still paying attention to your pulse, slowly exhale. What did you notice? As you took a breath in, you might have noticed a slight increase in the rate of your pulse and as you breathed out you might have noticed it slowing down. This is a great example of how your breath can modulate your heart rate. Cool, huh?!

We're going to learn how to use breathing to turn the calming switch on. To do this, we need to get in touch with our own natural

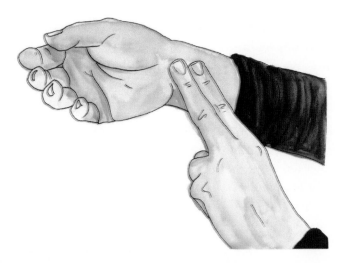

Finding your radial artery pulse

breathing rhythm, so first things first, notice what's happening right now. Go ahead and take a few breath cycles to tune in to your own natural breathing flow. What did you notice? How did you feel? Try it again, paying attention to any changes you notice with your unique breath pattern the second go round.

Our breathing patterns are transitory, always changing. You might have noticed differences the second time around. Just like with posture, so many of us have been told that we're breathing all wrong. That's just a bunch of bullshit if you ask me. If that's the case, I'm surprised any of us are still alive! Breathing shouldn't feel like a chore or make you worried about whether or not you're doing it well enough.

Anchor into your breath wherever and however it feels comfortable and safe in your body to do so. You'll soon become aware of how your own breath changes with certain contexts and circumstances, and the feelings associated with them. Once you gain an appreciation for this awareness, you can begin to manipulate your breath to a slower, softer and deeper breath to help modulate the pain response.

Now that you've taken a moment to witness what's normal for you, let's practice a form of breathing that is commonly taught: *focused* diaphragmatic breathing.

Focused diaphragmatic breathing pivots your awareness to the integrated sensations of your breath and your experience of your breath in your entire body. I say focused because all breathing is diaphragmatic breathing. We wouldn't be able to breathe without our diaphragm in the first place. If at any time this breathing exercise makes you uncomfortable, setting off a protective response, go back to your natural breathing rhythm. You can explore flowing between these two patterns if you'd like. Again, there are no rules. This is a time to be compassionately curious about your body.

Find a quiet place and take a comfortable sitting or lying-down position. At first, it might be easier to feel the expansiveness of the diaphragm and your breath while lying down, but eventually you'll practice your breath awareness in a variety of situations. Breathing is something you can take anywhere and use anytime, which is why it's one of my favorite tools to help turn down the neurological noise.

Place your hands on each side of your lower ribs. Settle in. Soften your shoulders, jaw and mouth. Gently close your eyes or keep them open, if you prefer.

As you take a deeper breath in, notice your belly and lower ribs rise and expand, a bit like a balloon. Feel the sensation of your ribs gently

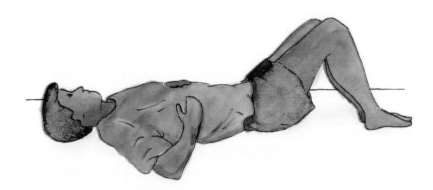

expanding into your hands and out towards the surface you're lying on.

You might find yourself trying hard to focus on this breathing thing, and it might feel different if you've never practiced this before. It's okay. You're learning something new, so cut yourself some slack if you don't get it right away. Accept what your body can do right now instead of forcing change. Forcing anything will create more resistance and tension in your body, which defeats the purpose of letting go.

After you've practiced paying attention to the sensations at your rib cage, let's add more awareness to the rest of your body.

THREE-POINT BREATH FOCUS

Place one hand on your belly and one hand at your heart. Settle into your natural breathing rhythm for a few breath cycles. When you're ready, imagine you're filling your whole torso with air, like you're filling a balloon in your belly. (Breathe a little into your belly, then your chest and lastly into your collar bones.) You can shift the order any way you'd like and choose a pace that feels good for you. Do this for a few breath cycles, observing how your breath and sensations at your belly, chest and collar bones change with every breath in and every breath out.

There are many other fun ways to manipulate your breathing, but for now, keep things simple. Just being aware of your breath with single-pointed focus is a great accomplishment.

BREATH WITH PELVIC AWARENESS

Get comfy. This would be a good time to invest in some pillows, blankets, or even a bolster (a long, thick and firm supportive cushion). Anything like that will be helpful for this exercise.

When starting out, it's useful to find a quiet space where you can focus on tuning in to how your body's feeling. Connecting with the pelvic floor is no easy task, especially if all you know down there is pain. With this exercise, we're going to explore sensations that you feel other than the pain. So, I recommend gifting yourself a few minutes of alone time. Maybe even pop on some of your favorite music, which may help your brain release its own pain-relieving chemicals.

Start by sitting with your back facing the bolster or pillows. Slowly lower yourself down to rest your back on top of the bolster.

Bring your feet together so the soles of your feet touch, allowing your knees to open out to the side. If this reclined posture is not

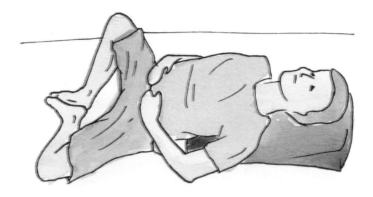

comfortable, feel free to try the same pose but without the bolster. If you feel like your legs are straining and inner thighs are too tight, use pillows for support underneath your knees.

This posture should feel comfortable. If it doesn't, adjust your posture in any way that you like or use more props. Everyone's got nerve sensors that have their own preferences, just like in the story of Goldilocks and the Three Bears. The point here is to recalibrate the nervous system, so if you're not feeling yummy in this shape, that would defeat the purpose. I love this restful pose because it allows spaciousness for the pelvis and hips, and the feedback you get from your hands on your belly deepens the awareness of the breath and pelvic-diaphragm synchrony.

As you take in your next breath, softly guide the breath into your lower ribs, belly and down into your pelvis. You may notice your belly soften as it expands, your sitz bones (the bony part of your butt that you sit on) broaden, and the pelvic floor muscles expand outward. Notice the sensations you feel around the area between the base of your penis and anus. If you're still having a hard time bringing awareness to your pelvic floor muscles, and it feels safe to do so, place your hand between the base of the penis and anus to tap into the subtle movement.

As you sink into your sensory experience, what other images, colors, or textures come to mind that help you reconnect with calmness here? As you breathe out, notice the sensations of the effortless change in direction as your chest, belly, and pelvic muscles draw back in towards the body.

You don't have to do this activity lying down on your back. You can tap into this awareness anywhere, anytime. Let your breath keep you grounded throughout the day. This is one way to create space in your cup so that it doesn't spill over with stress. You might notice the effects right away. Some days will be easier than others. Again, it all depends on how full your cup is to start. How would it feel to let go of instant gratification? Even when you think it's not working, keep at it because you're planting seeds for improvement, a neurological reset. Trust me, it gets easier the more you do it. The brain will eventually catch up and loosen the grip on danger, allowing mental and physical tensions to ease up.

This practice is about finding the balance between effort and ease. In the end, it will be more automatic and ingrained in your brain so you won't have to give it as much thought. The practice of tuning into your breath sensations allows you to check in on your physiological state of affairs at any time affording plenty of opportunities to water the seeds of those freshly planted neurological pathways. The mind and body are inseparable, so whether you're working on the physical or the mental aspects of pain, know that both will influence each other.

One more thing! Practice, practice, practice. It takes lots of practice and patience to strengthen neural connections. We'll be using breath awareness with other activities later on in this book.

NEED TO NOTICE

This type of breathing works best when you can recognize and bring awareness to your triggers. Start to note when, what, and where you tend to notice tension in your whole body, not just staying hyper-focused on your pelvis. If you're tensing or gripping your butt or belly throughout the day, notice if your pelvic floor muscles are joining in on the parade. To reiterate, tension is not a bad thing. There are many individuals who tense this and tense that, but who don't experience pain. Tension becomes bothersome when you don't like the experience you feel in your body. When that's the case, we need to shift this experience so you can begin to feel safe in your body again.

To help you notice that things are always changing, you'll need to first define your own body map and what the space surrounding it feels like. It's not uncommon to have the bits that hurt feel a bit weird, detached or fuzzy. It's often very difficult to even describe what it is that we're feeling and experiencing in our bodies when we're in pain. Sometimes it's helpful to use your imagination to express what you're feeling on the inside so that you can begin to regain a sense of self, using your own body to make changes to the neural underpinnings of pain.

Some questions you can ponder to help define the space in and around the bits that hurt.

If the parts of your body that hurt were...
A texture, what texture would they be?
- *What texture do you want them to feel like?*

A shape, what shape would they be?
- *What shape do you want them to be?*

A color, what color would they be?
- *What color would you like them to be?*

Made out of Playdough, what would happen as you molded it?
- *What would you want it to look like?*

Using your imagination to scan your body head-to-toe or toe-to-head will be useful to paint a picture of your embodied self. You can do this by following a brief audio-guided body scan exercise, which you can access here: https://bit.ly/2FlkT3E.

You can use your breath and body-scanning to play with the tension you feel in your body and mind at various times in your day. This will help you feel more in control of your body's reactions to various stressors.

Progressive muscle relaxation is another way you can approach gaining better control of how you feel in your body. The simplest way to help you understand this concept is for you to play a little game with me. Ready? (I'm assuming you said yes, so here we go.)

Make a fist with either hand. Squeeze tight. Allow the tension to in your hand to build up. Notice how the sensations in your hand change as you keep squeezing. How does the rest of your arm feel? What about your neck and shoulders? Oh, and don't forget to check in with your breath. Has your breathing changed at all? Now keeping all those areas in mind, begin to soften your hand just a little, a little bit more, a little bit more and finally let it all go. How did you go? Did you forget to think about your pain in that brief moment?

You have more control than you think over the tension in your body. Progressive muscle relaxation does just this. It allows you to experience tension in your body along with the experience of releasing and letting go.

So, how does this work? Just like you did with the body-scanning exercise, you can explore gently building up muscle tension in various parts of your body, for example by raising your eyebrows, smiling ear to ear, shrugging your shoulders, and yes, even tensing your pelvic muscles, all the while maintaining a soft, smooth, natural breathing pace. You'll soon begin to appreciate the change in sensations in your body by noticing how quickly the pressure and intensity you feel melt away when you let go voluntarily.

This is great practice to lessen the fear around tension and gain greater sense of control over your muscle function. It's not just about letting go and relaxing your pelvic muscles. It's impossible to completely relax them anyway. You wouldn't want to because you'd have poor control of your bodily fluids, if you catch my meaning! Motor control is about functional application for what you want to gain out of a particular activity. In the case of pelvic muscle function, it's important to practice building up tolerance to tissue tension. (If you need a reason, squeezing and letting go is important for sexual function!)

For more guidance, listen to this audio recording of progressive muscle relaxation here: https://bit.ly/2Qu6uc5.

A MIND FULL OF LESS

If we checked in with our mind every so often, we'd notice it's a bit of a free-for-all up there. Our thoughts running rampant all over the place. It's like shaking a snow globe and never putting it down. But imagine what it would feel like to put down the snow globe and watch things settle down for a bit so you could truly appreciate the picture inside. Quieting your mind will quiet your nervous system, but you don't have to run away to a monastery on a mountaintop to get a taste of this peace of mind. In short, you don't have to be perfect at zen.

Practicing mindfulness is actually practicing a mind full of less. Less attention to doing, running around and meditating on your pain. It's taking a moment to breathe and witness the good, the bad and the ugly from a zoomed-out point of view. Observing your mind in such a way will create space between you and your thoughts and feelings. This doesn't mean you sweep thoughts and feelings under the rug. Eventually, that would mean the crap piled up under there and became a mound of dirt. No ignoring it, then. This means you'll still experience your thoughts and feelings without getting swept up in the drama.

Dealing with pelvic pain can be overwhelming with countless doctor visits, tests, scans, treatments, etc. Oftentimes, you lose yourself in the chaos of it all. Well, it's time to put down that snow globe down and let the glitter settle. How? Through eavesdropping on your mind.

So, what *is* mindfulness? Mindfulness can be defined in many different ways depending on the source and context. For simplicity's sake, let's use the definition of a *state of being aware*[178] or just taking notice. For practical purposes, it means:

➤ Noticing what happens when you have pain
➤ Noticing when you're getting caught up in the storyline
➤ Being curious about all that the present moment has to offer you
➤ Noticing how your thoughts, feelings, pain, behavior/actions, and emotions influence each other
➤ Taking the opportunity to make choices that help you move closer towards the life you want to live.

PRACTICING MINDFULNESS WITH PELVIC PAIN

Practicing a mind full of less during times of stress and pain can help boost all your self-help efforts. (Although it's worth remembering these little practices during times of low stress and less pain, too, as it's not always easy to put new habits in place when the dial is already turned up.) This is a process of giving yourself more head space to be aware of and notice with curiosity all that surrounds the parts that hurt as well as everything in between. Noticing what's happening in your whole body can feel like safety in itself.

Let's try something right now. Set a timer for one minute. Stick out your thumb so it's in line with your field of vision. Stare at your thumb. Notice all the subtle nuances of your thumb like the color, temperature, size, texture, shape, feel and maybe even taste. Think long and hard about your thumb (not your penis). Come on now, keep that laser-like focus going for just a minute. Okay, now relax your concentration. What did you notice doing this activity? You may have noticed it was difficult to hold anything else in your mind other than your thumb, even if that experience was only fleeting. Now try this with a different part of your body, like your ear lobe.

Simple practices like the one you just did are enough to refine your neural responses. When you train your brain to shift focus, you hurt less.

SHIFTING YOUR FOCUS

Check in with your pelvis and the rest of your body throughout the day with a sense of compassionate curiosity. Get absorbed in what you notice without judgment or criticism. We tend to spend a lot of time and energy paying attention to experiences and labeling them as 'good', 'bad', 'painful', 'scary', 'pleasant', 'frustrating', etc. I encourage you to tap into your body throughout the day just as a silent observer. No need to get carried away in the narrative. Thoughts, sensations, and feelings are transient. If we can learn to be still with these experiences and resist less, the quicker they will pass, like clouds in the sky on a stormy day.

You could also think about this in terms of *clean* pain versus *dirty* pain, as coined by JoAnne Dahl and Tobias Lundgren in *Living Beyond Your Pain*.[179] Clean pain is the human experience of physical and emotional pain. Often, we don't have much control over what experiences we're dealt with in our lives. The mercurial sensations, feelings and emotions we're familiar with are normal responses during difficult times. Dirty pain is when spinning thoughts and exaggerated judgments muddy the sensory experience of pain. It's an added burden that causes suffering to ensue.

Research shows that being able to shift your attention in this way can influence areas of your brain related to pain sensitivity.[180] In other words, being better at delegating your attention can better help you manage and ease your pain.

As you purposefully and mindfully check in with yourself, focus your attention on the changing sensations you feel with movement, static postures, or breathing. Feel free to float your attention between any of these (or even shift your attention to and from particular areas of your body) in a non-judgmental way. Acknowledge any thoughts, feelings or associated emotions that come up for you, but then gently redirect your attention back to the sensations of the posture, movement, breath, etc.

With any sensations you notice, describe the quality and location of them (such as noting the texture, temperature, pressure, intensity, color, or stretch). Remember, you're connecting with your sensory experience for what it is and not as it appears. If you notice yourself getting carried away by the stories your mind tells you, know that this is completely normal. Noticing gives you the choice to change habits. Remember, your brain with its many complex neural connections and predictive capabilities is trying to make sense of your experience. And taking a wild guess, at best! This is not an entirely accurate measure of the health of your tissues.

Try not to get discouraged if you find yourself getting distracted and redirecting 100 times over. You should celebrate! This means you're getting better at catching yourself being distracted and becoming present in the moment. This constant redirection of your attention is the actual practice.

Try this exercise several times throughout the day. It doesn't have to be long or drawn out. It just has to be long enough to make it worthwhile, for you to pay attention and notice.

As you can imagine, this practice itself takes courage, persistence, and a willingness to 'go there.' The more you can be familiar with your autopilot habits, the better you can use strategies to change your experience with them.

When you first practice mindfulness, it's hard. I'm not here to lie to you. It'll take consistent practice to focus your attention on the present moment, even if that moment is painful.

Be aware of the thoughts that go on in your head during times of pain, allowing them to ebb and flow, but try not to react to them. It's natural to want to react to pain by tensing up or distracting yourself, but I encourage you to not do that. Instead, recognize how your body's feeling and observe it without changing a thing. Sometimes you've got to 'go into something to get out of it.' Sorta like a stuck drawer.

The more you can integrate this practice in your daily life, the more control you're going to have over how you feel and how your body reacts to certain situations. If you need help getting into the groove, check out these resources:

- ➤ Headspace (headspace.com)
- ➤ Curable (curablehealth.com)
- ➤ Calm (calm.com)
- ➤ Insight Timer (insighttimer.com)
- ➤ Mindfulness Meditation for Pain Relief (soundstrue.com/products/mindfulness-meditation-for-pain-relief)
- ➤ Buddhify (buddhify.com)
- ➤ HeartMath (heartmath.com)

DISTRACTION IS YOUR FRIEND

Wait a sec. Didn't I just get done telling you how important it was to be present in the moment? Uh-huh, I did. But that doesn't mean distraction doesn't have its own benefits. Indeed, they aren't mutually exclusive at all. Distraction is a form of awareness on something other than your pain. Similar to the exercise on shifting your focus, distraction disrupts pain neurotags.[181] Distractions are free and have no side effects. They might just be the best pain relievers out there!

Of course, there's a catch! (There's no silver bullet, remember.) Distractions need to be meaningful and worthwhile, possibly even worth experiencing a little bit of discomfort alongside them. Avoiding activities that have previously been painful doesn't allow for the opportunity to experience them with less pain. This reinforces your expectation that it will continue to hurt whenever you engage in that activity.[182] [183] Attending to pain in an acute situation is protective and necessary for survival. Heck, you'd want to know if you stepped on a nail, wouldn't you? But attending to pain in a chronic situation no longer serves its purpose. In fact, it gets in the way of you living your life to the fullest. So, it's a balance between not enough attention versus too much attention. This varies by individual and by the context in which you find yourself.

USE YOUR SENSES

Sometimes just being aware of what's happening outside and inside of your body can be grounding, especially if you can't 'get out of your head.' Whenever you feel like you're on the verge of screaming "I just can't take it anymore," pause, pat yourself on the back for noticing, and intentionally tap into your five senses. You can do this activity anywhere, anytime.

I encourage techniques like these often, even practicing them when you're not in distress. Think about it this way. You're adding to your storeroom of resilience, so that when the stakes rise, you've got enough in reserve to tap into and use. Practice helps build self-regulation and mental flexibility.

Here's how it goes:
- ➤ Name **five** things you can see right now
- ➤ Feel **four** things you can touch
- ➤ Listen to **three** things you can hear
- ➤ Sniff **two** things you can smell
- ➤ Savor **one** thing you can taste.

Get in touch with your sensory experience instead of the narrative. This exercise can be especially helpful to get a handle on the mind chatter when you feel a flare-up coming on. It helps you to anchor down while allowing yourself to *feel* in the present moment even when it's painful.

Other mindful-like practices that you could explore:

> **Walking** – Take a walk outside for five minutes. Purposefully pay attention to what it is that you're noticing and, when you're done, take a moment to notice what you noticed. Maybe you felt a breeze brush up against your skin, your feet grounded with the earth, or how the temperature on your body changed as you passed sunnier versus shadier areas.

> **Yoga** – It's not just for chicks and yogis. NFL players and the military have adopted yoga as part of their regular training routine. Go figure! Yoga helps reduce stress, pain, anxiety and improves mobility, and agility.[184] [185] [186] Side effects of feeling better? Improved sexual health and wellbeing!

> **Tai chi and Qigong** – Like yoga, these are centuries-old mind-body practices that involve mental focus and awareness using certain movements, body postures and breathing. They can help reduce pain and stress while improving overall mood and quality of life.[187]

> **Dancing** – Oh yeah, shake it! Not only is it a good cardio workout, but you get all the feel-good benefits too. Go ahead, bust out that happy dance even if you're faking it.

On the subject of movement, let's continue on to some physical practices.

CHAPTER 7

PLEASURE-HUNTING!

Get your map out because we're going pleasure-hunting! Sometimes, people with pelvic pain have been focused on pain for so long that they forget what it feels like to experience anything positive in their body or in some cases even in their life. Together, we'll explore movements, stretches, and safe touch to reconnect you with a sense of feeling good in your body and yourself.

Before reading on any further, take a moment to reflect on this question:

What does feeling good look like for you?

There's a bunch of studies that propose changes take place in areas of the brain dedicated to receiving sensory information from the body, and this contributes to the perpetuation and increased intensity of ongoing pain.[188] [189] Adaptations like these can make the bits of you that hurt feel 'weird', 'alien', and disconnected from the rest of your body. There's not enough evidence to support whether or not this 'reorganization' of the nervous system is the *cause* of perpetual pain, but it does show us that pain involves a multitude of complex factors throughout the systems of the body and mind, not just in your tissues. Again, great defense mechanism in the short term, but not so helpful in the long term. Put briefly, the same system built to *protect* you keeps pain on repeat (regardless of actual tissue damage or harm).

Okay, biology briefing over. I've already talked your ear off about this in previous chapters. Suffice to say, just because your nerves have gone *haywire*, it doesn't mean you're a lost cause. Your nerve sensors are constantly changing and adapting, and can 'rewire', which means you can feel calmer and safer in your body to move, sit, play, touch, and get back to doing the things you love. Knowing that your nervous system and other bodily systems adapt to protect you gives you the opportunity to work with your body and brain in fun and creative ways that help re-establish harmony within your nervous system and your life.

One way to do this is to use sensory integration techniques to restore healthy tolerance to touch, movement, and yes, even activities like sex.

So, what is sensory integration? Simply put, this means using all five senses to provide multiple kinds of 'feel good' or at least less threatening inputs to alter the outputs. I say this simply, but in reality the inputs and outputs are working in tandem and simultaneously, influencing each other moment by moment.

We're going to use sensory input in a variety of ways to change your relationship with your current experience by facilitating your own neural processes. This allows your own neural processes to adapt in response to safe and pleasurable sensory cues. In fact, without you knowing it, a lot of the strategies already discussed earlier in this book were sensory integration practices. To get a little more physical, in this section, you're going explore movement, stretching, different postures and shapes, then finish up with some hand-y work.

PACING YOURSELF

Probably the most counterproductive decision you can make when in pain is to stop doing what you love. Why? Because a wheel in motion, even going really slowly, is easier to speed up again than if you've completely stopped. Instead of closing yourself off from the world for fear of a flare-up, keep some momentum in your social life and have a wee bit of fun. What does fun look like for you? When was the last time you had a good time?

There's good evidence to support that having a healthy social web helps strengthen your immune system and decreases pain sensitivity.[190] [191] [192] When you're not alone and you have a support system in place, whether that is family, friends, support groups, journaling, counselors, meditation, therapists, furry pals, wellness providers, pretty much anything you want, you're better able to get through those crummy days, but also more likely to celebrate your progress on the good ones.

Aside from having the right people in your life, the key to getting back into the swing of things is spoon-feeding. Activities like sex, food, drinking, exercising, sitting, and working all require dosing so that you minimize your risk of temper tantrums. Whoops, I mean flare-ups! Do you remember the overflowing cup activity I had you reflect on earlier? This would be a good time to pull that out again because the activities that you want to make room for in your cup will require some space in there. When you're in pain, the protective systems are amped up and the alarm bells keep ringing, which can make it difficult to enjoy life. Rest assured there is still a way to self-soothe your nervous system one spoonful at a time.

1. Start with one activity that you really want to do more of (i.e. sex, driving, sitting, standing, reading, masturbating, walking, running, hiking, gym time, going to the movies, you get the idea).

2. Find your baseline. How much of that activity can you do without a flare-up?

3. Start small and build up. Incrementally increase your exposure to the activity you choose and be consistent. It's important to plan your baseline increases in advance, so pencil them into your day.

Remember, you're creating new familiarity, not replaying the pain song. The more positive experiences you can have with a certain activity that is painful, the more you begin to break down the neural connections and negative predictions associated with that experience.

Finding your baseline might be tricky at first, so to increase your chances of having a positive experience, let's start with some motor imagery. Imagining yourself doing an activity can be just as good as actually doing it and has been shown to be an effective treatment strategy for pain.[193] Of course, the eventual goal would be to be able to do the activity you want. Just thinking about it won't magically translate into function, although it's a good start to lessen the threat around activities you're afraid to do. When you imagine doing a movement, you activate similar motor areas in the brain that light up during actual execution of that movement.[194] Sorta like an architect who imagines the design of a building in their mind before entering the details in a computer and then manages the construction project. You're going be your own body's architect, but before you call your construction crew, the blueprints have to be ready.

Take a moment to use your imagination to create a plan for an activity that you want to get back to doing. Like an athlete, visualize the play-by-play in your head. Add in different scenarios, environments, contexts, etc.

One challenge that might hinder your progress is that the thought of doing something can make you cringe, like the thought of having your ball-sack bouncing back and forth during sex. If you've got pain in your testicles, I'm sure this thought has crossed your mind many times. Here's another example you might know well. Do you experience pain with sitting? Like many people in your situation, sitting can be a challenge, so let's start your visualization there.

As far as it's possible for you, settle into a comfortable position. Then imagine yourself sitting on a firm surface. Notice how your body feels with this image in your mind. Did your breathing change? How about muscle tension? What thoughts popped up? Did your pain increase? If yes, let's back up the challenge a bit.

Imagine sitting on a softer surface or maybe your favorite recliner. Maybe you imagine sitting in your favorite coffee shop, relaxing in a beach chair with your toes in the sand or eating lunch on your favorite hiking trail. Your imagination can even take you to the moon and back. How about that?! Gotta love the power of the mind.

Once you've landed in that sweet spot (with little to no pain or protection elicited), you've found your starting point. From here, you slowly and consistently turn up the challenge. You continue to do this until you can imagine sitting on a cactus without a protective pain response. Okay, I'll admit, maybe that's a bit extreme, but you get the point here. You want to be able to imagine sitting or doing any activity of your choosing with little to no protective response when you hold that image in your mind.

Once you've conquered that challenge, it's time to up the ante. Take

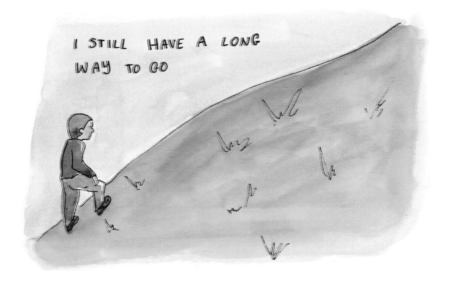

this out into the real world. You would start in the same incremental fashion as described above. Find the easiest starting point (like sitting on the comfiest chair possible even if it's for 10 seconds to start) and build up from there, daily. Realistically, you're probably sitting for more than 10 seconds a day, but the goal here is to carve out time purposefully and intentionally to pay attention, notice the sensations in your body, practice your mindfulness skills, build up tissue tolerance, and gather evidence for feeling 'good' or at least less crappy.

As you increase your acquaintance with those activities that were once 'forbidden,' it's common to experience some discomfort. Don't give up. Stay consistent. Remember, you might be 'sore but you're safe.' You can add some playfulness to this game by taking pictures of yourself doing these activities so that you can brag to your friends or therapist, and look back at these pictures to remind yourself of how far you've come. You can also drop notes into your 'win jar' and reflect on them at the end of the day, week, or month. The more we can positively reinforce safety and confidence in your body and your life, the more momentum we gather to move you forward on your recovery.

It's not uncommon for you to want to push yourself further too quickly as you start feeling better, but I wouldn't recommend it. We'd

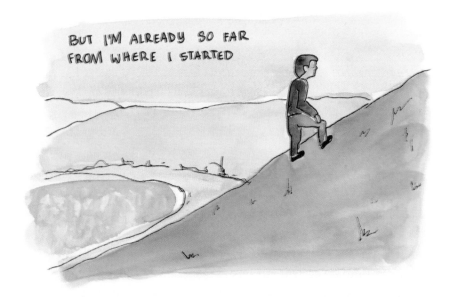

like to decrease your chances of having an unpleasant experience with these activities, but that's not always possible. You can always dial back down should you feel that you've pushed it too fast, too soon.

Other ways to supercharge your experience and success is to combine these activities with your favorite music to get you motivated and pumped. C'mon, we've all got our favorite jams that make us groove no matter where we're at. Or maybe you have a buddy who knows how to make you laugh. Or a favorite scent that reminds you of the 'good times'. However you achieve the dopamine hit, if it evokes feeling good, it'll build up stronger neural connections for feeling safe in your body with that activity.

Strategies like the one just mentioned can be applied to just about anything, even sexy time. Again, this isn't a one-size-fits-all approach. The mission is to 'nudge to but not through,' when you're building up your physical and mental resilience and flexibility.

Pacing principles work well when you can control your environment, but there will be times where pacing isn't going to be possible. So, how flexible are you in any given situation? Work with your pain care team to customize a plan to fit your unique needs.

And remember, if you flare-up, don't freak out.

FLARE-UP PLAN

Ever veered a little out of your lane on the highway and gotten a wake-up call by the rumble strips? Creating a flare-up plan is sorta like that, a friendly nudge to help you get back into your lane. I'm sure you would agree that it would be ah-mazing if you could avoid flare-ups altogether, but we need to be realistic, sometimes that's just not possible. Life's unpredictable.

Awareness will play a role here too. Much of pain is driven by subconscious processes and sometimes your body will give off subtle signs that distress is brewing. Again, things like tension in other parts of your body, breathing changes, mood changes, fatigue, bladder grumpiness, nervous twitching, etc. When identifying your triggers earlier on, you might have noticed that these messages are present in certain situations or contexts more than others and at varying intensities. Being aware of any 'pre-sensations' or other visceral responses will be helpful to 'put out the fire' sooner than later. It's much easier to extinguish a bonfire than it is to tame a forest fire.

In case you need to pull the fire alarm and grab the fire extinguisher, remember the acronym PASS.

Pause
Assess
'Sore but safe' mantra
Seek safety

Let's break it down.

Pause to breathe. Reorient your attention on your breath. Notice your breath sensations. Then, intentionally steer your breath slow and steady.

Assess your current situation. Is this situation really dangerous? To my body? To me as person? To my lifestyle?

'Sore but safe' mantra. Reassure yourself by remembering that these sensations do not equate to tissue damage.

Seek safety. You know your body best. What can you do to help yourself feel safe in your body in this moment?

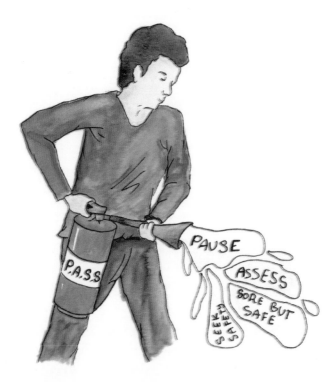

Sometimes it can be helpful to have this written down somewhere easily accessible or in a place where you'll remember to check it. Make a list of items that can help you redirect and land your plane so you can feel grounded in your body in the moment. The most useful and accessible tool – anytime, anyplace – is your breath. You can also phone a friend, go for a walk, stretch, journal or use several of the suggested strategies from this book or those from your own experiences, which are always the best!

Keep in mind, although you're experiencing more sensitivity than usual, it doesn't mean you're back at square one. Flare-ups are part of the process, and the less you resist or fear them, the better off you'll be.

You might have to modify some activities or make fewer commitments, but you will continue to move forward. Do gentle exercise and movements. Take any necessary medication – if possible, just in the short term. Add in purposeful and meaningful rest, whatever 'rest' may look like for you. And maybe hardest of all, stay positive.

Then, slowly and gradually build things back up.

MOTION IS LOTION

Speaking of gentle movements, let's moooove. Take a break from reading and refresh your brain and tissues with some movement. As they say, 'motion is lotion.' So, get up, move around, wiggle your butt, stretch your arms up towards the sky, twist like a washing machine, or dance around like a monkey. What you do is up to you, but get movin'.

Hopefully that quick refresher put some fresh, oxygenated blood into tissues that needed some lovin'! It's not uncommon for any of us to experience muscle tightness or joint stiffness when we've been sitting too long, like after a long car ride or being absorbed in a book for hours! Messages from nerve sensors influenced by neurochemicals and changes in tissue blood flow alert your brain to get you to move, so naturally you might find yourself fidgeting in your seat or getting up to take a nice big stretch, which usually makes the achy, stiff feelings go away. It's a great way to promote necessary nourishment to your tissues so they don't get cranky. Some pain experiences can be perpetuated by postural habits, misuse or disuse of tissues. In persistent pain, however, we know that it's far more complex than this, even though what I've just described could be *one* of many contributing factors.

Hang on to your *unmentionables* because I'm about to challenge your thoughts about muscle tightness and joint stiffness. Muscle tightness and joint stiffness have less to do with actual changes in muscle and joint structure and probably more to do with adaptations in your nervous system (cue halting screech of car brakes). Just think about this for a sec. If you've ever stretched anything before, you know that the gains you feel immediately after don't last forever. Some days you're able to bend forward and touch your toes, other days not. If stretching or not stretching tissues actually made long-term structural changes to your muscles and joints, wouldn't these changes presumably last forever? You might argue that it depends on how long and how frequently you're stretching that makes the difference. Living tissues constantly adapt and change based on tissue demands and within a context. Nothing remains fixed or static. Now for the amazing part. Did you know that you can gain more flexibility with *resistance training* than passive stretching?[195] So, are you even permanently changing the structure of your muscles when stretching? Some say yes and some say no. You could spend a lifetime studying the science behind stretching and still not have a conclusive answer! (Yup, some people dedicate their lives to this research!)

The nitty gritty details behind stretching are beyond the scope of this book. There's still much we don't know on this topic that has yet be discovered. The mysteries of the human body are beautifully complex, miraculous and amazing! In the next few paragraphs, I would like to share what I understand and have learned from scouring the literature on this topic.

Most likely, both sensory and mechanical mechanisms are involved when it comes to the perceived after-effects of stretching. Some human and animal studies[196] [197] [198] [199] suggest that changes in muscle flexibility might be due to temporary changes in the viscoelastic properties of the tissues being loaded. Living tissues show both viscous and elastic behavior. *Viscous* meaning adapting characteristics of a liquid-like behavior (gooey, syrupy) and elastic meaning returning back to its original shape once tension is removed (like the tension from a stretch). One good way to explain this concept is thinking about coconut oil. In a jar, coconut oil is thick, hard, and solid. Add a little heat to it, and it transforms right before your eyes into a different form. Remove the heat, and watch it turn back to solid again. Although the texture of coconut oil changes under different environments, it never loses its essence of being coconut oil. Viscoelastic behavior in living tissues depends on the type of internal and external stressors applied to tissues, speed and time that the stress is applied, genetic variability, psychosocial context in which the load is applied, and much more.

Most likely, the changes in sensation, range of motion, and performance that you feel after you do a stretch have to do with sensory tolerance changes rather than actual structural tissue changes like tissue lengthening.[200] [201] [202] [203] [204] A muscle's job is to resist change. Initially, muscle resistance to change is high, but with increasing or repetitive load application, the resistance to stress (change) becomes less over time.[205] How this occurs depends on the individual's make-up variances, their experiences, the importance of an activity, function of the body part involved, neural influence, consciousness, and more.

Here's a study that'll make you think... Researchers looked at hamstring stretch (non-involved leg) in 15 people undergoing selective knee surgery. They found that hamstring stretch was greatest while under anesthesia, suggesting that neural influences are at play when it comes to range of motion and flexibility.[206] Tissue stretch perception relies on specialized mechanoreceptors that detect proprioceptive input and report this information to the brain. The brain influences this process at the same time, so input and output are simultaneously influencing one another.

Changes in range of motion, performance, flexibility, or how you feel in your body are most likely due to both muscle composition changes (that are load-dependent, though how much load is yet to be determined) and neural adaptations. Feelings of tightness and stiffness is a conscious perception driven by numerous subconscious neurocognitive processes very much like pain. By slapping a label and accepting mainstream ways of thinking about muscles as being 'shortened' or 'overstretched' and often blamed for pain or 'poor posture,' we oversimplify the complexities of muscle function, which is actually living, adaptable tissue.

Evidence suggests that adaptive changes in actual muscle length from acute, passive stretching is slim.[207] [208] A famous research paper by Harvey and colleagues in 2017 shocked many of us in the physical therapy world. Let me explain why. These researchers gathered, reviewed and analyzed a ton of research studies on the topic of stretching to prevent and treat contractures. To clarify terms, the word contracture is derived from the Latin term *contractura* which means to 'draw together.'[209] If you look up the definition of a contracture on the internet, you'll probably read a definition similar to "a shortening of muscles, tendons, or other tissues producing joint deformity."[210] They studied more than 1400 participants collectively and found that stretching didn't work for people with contractures due to either neurological or non-neurological conditions. A measly 1-2 degrees change in range of motion, at most, was seen across the board![211] That's like trying to salt your food with one grain of salt. It won't make a difference for your taste buds.

But wait, there's more! The amount of time spent stretching didn't matter either. The average difference made with stretching for every 1 hour logged was 0 degrees, yup, 0 degrees.[212] Some study participants even spent hundreds of hours stretching in a splint. That's a lot of work for so little return. One would assume, if tissues were structurally shortened, tightened, or contracted, prolonged stretching would put tissues back to health. Unfortunately, this piece of research showed contrary to popular belief.

Even stretching other parts of your body can result in range of motion changes in the parts that feel tight, stiff and stubborn![213] In other words, it's not just the sensory messages coming from your tissues that make you feel stiff, tight, or loosey goosey.

In a 2017 study, scientists discovered that *feelings* of stiffness in the lower back have little to do with actual structural changes in the back when back stiffness and biomechanics were formally measured. In fact, those who reported lower back pain and stiffness actually overestimated the amount of force applied to their back and noticed even the tiniest change in force compared to those without lower back pain.[214] Another interesting takeaway from this article is that the addition of an auditory stimulus in combination with applied force to the back also changed the perception of what participants felt (overestimation of force). This further suggests that *feelings* of stiffness are multisensory and that other senses (what you hear, taste, touch, see and smell) influence the perception of bodily sensations and can trigger the need for protection or safety. Again, it all depends on the context, your thoughts, beliefs, previous experiences, environment, lessons and so on.

When you're not in pain, you probably don't even pay attention to the subtle movements and nuances of the frequent position changes and fidgeting that take place. Tissues need oxygen and movement helps with just that. Herein lies the problem. You're experiencing pain, and pain makes you pay very close attention. Pain changes your physiology and how you act in order to seek protection. Muscles will tense to protect sensitive tissues or in response to an emotionally triggering or stressful event. Again, all normal effects of experiencing pain. This heightened protection and attention that pain demands of you can really magnify the painful bits of your body so that even the slightest changes in your body are detected and protected, as we see in the study just mentioned.

Some guys report that it feels like 'guitar strings' down there. Tight, tense, and super uncomfortable. Maybe you can relate? Although these feelings are concerning and alarming, pain, muscle tightness, and stiffness often go together like cookies and cream. Altered bodily sensations are protective responses of a hyper-alert nervous system. And just like pain, sensations have the ability to change and feel safe again. Muscles don't actually shorten and knot up like guitar strings, although it sure can feel like it sometimes!

Now, this doesn't mean that stretching as a movement option isn't helpful. There are many ways to move and many ways to define stretching depending on the outcomes you're seeking. For the purposes of this book, stretching can be anything that changes the tensile load applied to your tissues and gets you to move, nourishing your tissues. The best part? You get to choose what that is for you. Whether you're actively engaging your body in slow repetitive movements, bouncing around or using a strap to reach your max, whatever your flavor, know that load is an important determinant for all your tissues to adapt, tolerate varying demands with activity, and build strength and resilience.[215]

Traditionally, you might've thought or been taught that muscles need to relax in order to 'stretch'. By now, you've gotten the hint that this isn't necessarily the case. Besides, stretching is a physical activity that gets you to move and is a great way to use your body to manipulate sensory information that will influence the protective processes of your nervous system and promote blood flow to tissues that are thirsty. Add in a sprinkle of mindful awareness, a drizzle of slow breathing, and top it off with your favorite music and you've got yourself a delightful safety sundae!

MOVEMENT SNACKS

Up next, you get to explore your body with some of my favorite shapes that we'll call movement snacks.

With any new physical activity regimen, there's a learning curve, so be sure to follow the pacing tips discussed earlier to find your preferred intensity and frequency. Some days it might feel easier; other days you might just feel like the tin man. Not a problem, though, because just like pain, it's a protective response. And that means it's changeable. Trust your body and learn to listen to it. It's normal to feel changes with pressure, stretch, and intensity when exploring how your body moves. Notice these changes as you move in and out of the various shapes and postures. You know the 'it's a good kinda hurt' feeling? That's okay. But if it doesn't feel right, then ease up or change things a bit. Maybe you need to modify your position, slow your breath, soften into the movement, or use props like pillows, blankets, blocks, straps, or whatever clever tools you find lying around your house, as long as they feel yummy when you use them.

The bottom line here is to tailor what you do and use to your body and your specific needs. Be curious with your exploration as if you suddenly found yourself in a pitch-dark room and needed to feel your way out stealthily. Do it with purpose and a sense of curiosity. Running frantically in a dark room full of unknown objects doesn't sound like a bright idea, right? The more purposeful and mindful you are of your movements, the less cautious your nervous system will be. Also, do an audit of how you feel in your body both before and after each activity. Take time to notice any changes you might feel. Again, this awareness of your 'embodied self' will help to recalibrate the nervous system creating a sense of safety and control in how you feel. The 'no pain, no gain' concept doesn't apply, so don't try to be macho. More is not always necessary to feel better.

As far as a 'protocol' goes, there isn't one. How many times you should be doing this or that is entirely up to you. There's really no right or wrong, good or bad. They are all experiences and learning opportunities. Use the pacing tips mentioned earlier and collaborate with your wellness team to find the right ingredients for your secret sauce if you need more help troubleshooting. Although there are no 'rules,' know that change does take time and that consistency with any practice influences progress. So, before you throw in the towel, ask yourself: did I really give it a chance?

The following shapes and movements are some of my go-to favorites. The purpose is to introduce novel and non-threatening sensory information to your nervous system. It's not about alignment or looking perfect in any one posture. It's more about noticing the change in sensations with pressure, stretch and intensity as you explore each posture with dynamic movements and static shapes. That being said it would be helpful to do a quick mind and body scan first to check in with yourself and get a sense of how your mind and body feel right now. The link to the guided audio can be found in the last chapter. Again, these are just suggestions, not rules. If it feels yummy, do more of that!

Oh, and as a bonus, you'll nourish your tissues. Motion is lotion... literally. Movement produces lubricin, a protein that makes your tissues slide and glide much more easily.[216] Just think what sex would feel like if there wasn't any lubrication compared to how it feels when there is. With these movements, you'll also be giving your nerves a nice stretch (and a drink, since nerves have their own blood supply and fluid for sliding and gliding), or tying in some pelvic neurodynamics, if you want to know the big fancy words for it.

One more suggestion, if you find yourself in a shape or movement that is initially uncomfortable or unpleasant, check in with your body and mind to notice the reactions to those feelings. You might notice muscle guarding or tension, specific thoughts, changes in range of motion or changes in your breathing. Are you willing to experience what would happen if you allowed your body to soften into the discomfort? How would that change your experience?

MELTING HEART

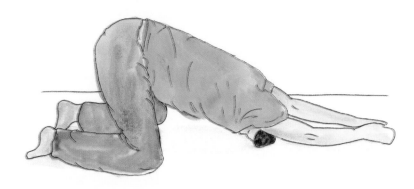

Come on to all fours. (This is sometimes referred to as table-top position.) Slowly walk your arms forward, lowering the top of your forehead and chest down towards the ground. Hips over your knees. Pause here for 5-10 breaths. Add a blanket under your forehead or knees for comfort if needed. You can also explore swaying your hips side to side, up and down, moving your arms over to one side and then the other. Notice the change in sensations as you explore this shape.

LETTING GO

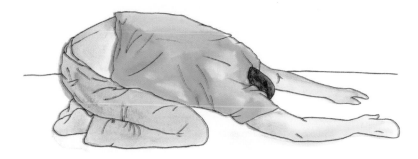

For you yoga fans out there, you might know this restorative posture as child's pose. Starting in the table-top position, sink your hips back towards your heels and stretch your arms forward. Rest your forehead on the ground or onto a blanket or even a bolster or pillow if this is accessible to you. Explore with the position of your knees, how does it feel to have them wide apart? Closer together? Feet together? Feet apart? Hands out in front or behind you? Walk your hands to the right. What does that feel like? Walk your hands to the left. How does that feel instead? Notice the change in sensations as you explore this shape.

CAT-COW

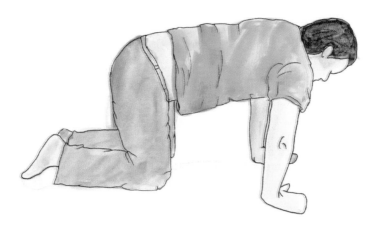

Here you're going to explore with curling and arching and your spine. First, begin in a neutral table-top position (on your hands and knees). On your next out-breath, gently press your palms into the ground, round

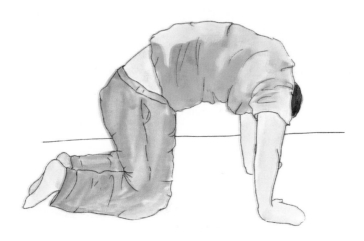

your back into a c-shape, tuck in your pelvis and let your head hang as if you were energetically drawing your nose towards your tailbone. Pause for a few breaths here to appreciate any sensations you might feel, then slowly come back to your neutral table-top position. Feel free to move back and forth between these two positions noticing changes in pressure, stretch and intensity in the sensations you feel. Combine this movement with your own natural, comfortable breath pace.

Next, explore arching your back. Returning back to table-top position, on your next in-breath, extend your tailbone out and lengthen your chest up towards the ceiling. This movement doesn't have to be particularly big. Do what feels right for your body. Explore with your head and neck. What does it feel like if you look straight ahead? What does it feel like if you lift your head slightly to look up? Visualize an energetic lengthening of your spine between the tailbone and the crown of your head. Play with moving back and forth between spine neutral and spine arching. Combine this movement with your own natural, comfortable breath pace.

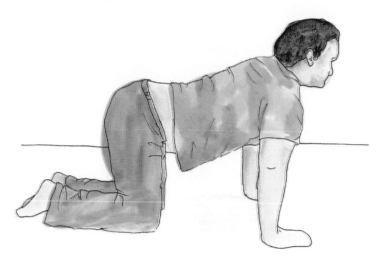

Ready to pull it all together? Play with alternating between the rounding and arching movements. A breath suggestion here is to inhale as you arch and exhale as you round your back. Notice the change in sensations you feel as you transition in and out of these shapes. Explore with smaller or larger extensions if that calls to you. Heck, you can even 'wag your tail,' moving your hips side to side and see what that feels like.

If your wrists feel cranky in this shape, experiment with making fists, using extra padding under your palms, or even placing your hands on some dumbbells. Cushion under the knees for comfort, if needed. You don't have to do this on your hands and knees either. Explore this movement sitting and standing. Notice the differences between doing it on hands and knees versus sitting versus standing. Adding movement with sitting can also be a helpful distraction especially if you experience pain with sitting. The key is giving some other parts of your body some love. Noticing sensations other than what is going on with the parts that hurt. When was the last time you checked in with your left earlobe? You won't know unless you try.

SEATED BOUND ANGLE

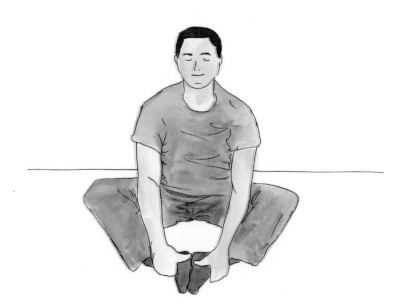

Take an easy seat. Be curious with what it feels like to have nothing under your bum versus propping your hips up with blankets, blocks, bolster, pillow, etc. Once you find your preference, bring the soles of your feet to touch. Hands can be resting in your thighs, wrapped around your feet, or propped behind you. Take a few breaths here and just notice how this shape serves you. With a curious intention, gently and slowly move your knees up and down, like a butterfly flapping its wings. What would it feel like to stretch one leg out straight? What about the other side? Sitting up tall or slouched? How does your right side feel compared to the left? This would also be a nice opportunity to try cat-cow in a different way. Again, you're just noticing with compassionate curiosity.

Another version of this shape that you could play around with is lying on your back with the soles of your feet touching. In either one of these postures, you could add pillows under the knees for comfort or just for the heck of it!

C-SHAPE

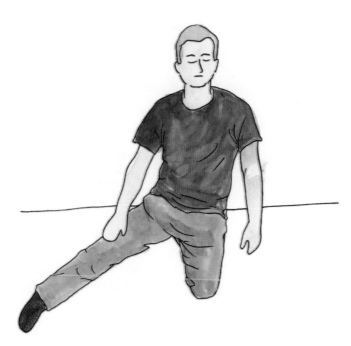

Begin in a tall kneeling position. Add a blanket under the knees for comfort if needed. Slowly extend one leg out the side, as shown in the picture above. If this already feels yummy, feel free to absorb yourself in the experience just as you are. If you're looking to spice things up a bit, on your next in-breath, raise your arms towards the ceiling. As you breathe out, simultaneously slide one arm down the extended leg and reach the other arm over your head or straight up towards the ceiling. Pause for a few breaths. Again, explore how these shapes feel for you. Notice the change in pressure, stretch and intensity that you may feel. Maybe you want to flow back and forth between raising both your arms up towards the ceiling and side bending into the c-shape. Sky's the limit with creativity here.

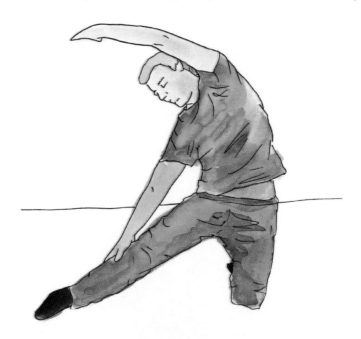

AIR SQUAT

Start by lying on your back. Take a moment to settle into your breath wherever that's most comfortable for you. Notice the sensations of your body just lying here. Then when you're ready, pull both knees toward your chest. Widen your knees apart as far as you feel safe and comfortable to do so. You may feel a sensation in the inner groin as you stretch tissues.

As you're breathing, see if you can soften your neck, shoulders, pelvic muscles, lower back, belly, and buttock muscles with every breath in and as you breath out. As you breathe in, notice a gentle expansion of

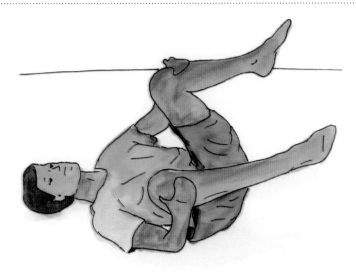

your pelvic floor muscles and visualize broadening of your sitz bones. Notice how it feels to be in this shape. Are you using all your might or hanging out with ease? What would it feel like to rock side to side? Forward and back?

If you find it hard to soften your body while keeping your knees up, rest your feet up on a wall for added support, or extend your legs

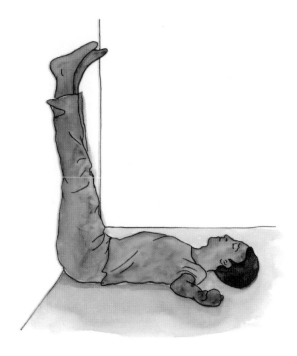

straight up the wall. With feet or legs supported on the wall, you can also experiment with some pelvic muscle coordination exercises by doing some 'reverse Kegels.'

REVERSE KEGELS

Performing a reverse Kegel is like letting out a fart or having a bowel movement. Instead of intentionally contracting, you're intentionally engaging your muscles in the opposite direction.

Close your eyes for a moment and notice any sensations in the pelvis, even if they're uncomfortable and painful, see if you are willing to explore and go into these sensations rather that resist or avoid. Remember, *clean* pain versus *dirty* pain? See if you can be with the sensations and not the storyline.

Next, pretend like you want to stencil the shape of your pelvis on a piece of paper underneath you or the surface you're sitting or lying on. What would it look like? Take a slightly deeper belly breath in. As you breathe out, gently let go of the tension around your anus as if you were trying to pass gas. (Sometimes you might actually fart and that's okay. Everyone farts.) You should feel a subtle bulge of your anus.

On your next breath out, focus on the front. The same technique applies but this time you're focusing on letting go of tension around the penis and testicles as if you were trying to pee.

Practice this technique several times, synchronizing it with your breath. Alternate between the front and the back. No need to hulk it here! This is a subtle awareness activity.

ASS TO GRASS

Start by standing with your feet wide apart and toes slightly pointed out to the side. Slowly stick your butt out and lower yourself towards the floor. Ease into this shape. You shouldn't feel like you're straining to hold yourself up. Take a few conscious breaths here. As you breathe, see if you can notice a gentle expansion of your diaphragm and visualize a widening of your sitz bones. Stand up and repeat.

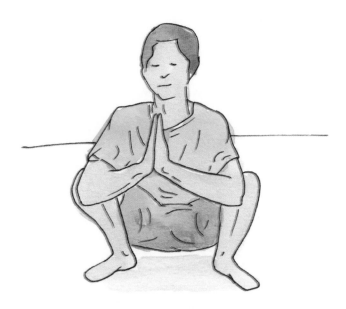

If balance is an issue, feel free to lean your back up against a wall for added support or lie down on your back with your knees wide apart. Hug them to your chest like in the modified air squat. If your hips or knees just don't feel comfortable in this position, try adjusting the width of your knees and orientation of your feet. You can also add a bolster, yoga block, or pillows under your sitz bones. If you find your heels aren't touching the floor, use a rolled-up yoga mat, towel, or half foam roller under your heels. If this shape feels comfortable for you, explore lifting your butt up a little and coming back down into the shape. You can also plant both palms down on the ground as if they were glued to the floor and lift your hips into the air, then come back down into the shape. Notice the change in sensations as you explore.

PRESS-UP

Start by lying front down on your belly. Slide your elbows to your sides and roll your shoulders back and away from your ears. Let your shoulders feel heavy and broad. Soften your lower back, butt cheeks and legs. As you take a comfortable breath in, straighten your arms and gently extend your back as you press yourself up. Allow gravity to take it from

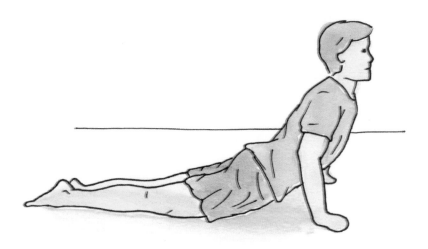

here as you melt into this shape for a few breath counts. Where does your body feel at ease? What areas feel more like a struggle? What are you noticing?

If extending your arms completely straight isn't accessible for you right now, try propping yourself onto your forearms instead. Use your breath to flow in and out of these positions, feeling the changes in pressure, intensity and stretch. Notice the sensations in the front of your body versus the back of your body. How do you feel afterwards?

FRONT THIGH STRETCH

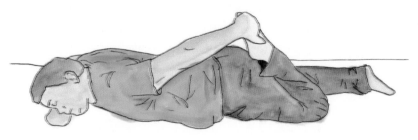

While lying on your belly, make a pillow with one of your forearms. Use the other hand to reach back for your foot and slowly guide your heel towards your butt. A strap comes in handy here if you find it challenging to reach back for your foot. While using a strap or your hand,

explore the sensations of lying flat on your belly versus propping yourself up on your forearm like in the picture below.

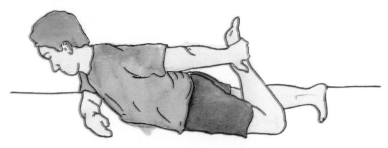

Move in and out of these postures and notice the different sensations as they wax and wane with each repetition. Maybe reaching back
for both feet is accessible for you today. Layer on the synchrony of your
breathing as you flow through the different movements or just hanging
out. Don't forget to explore the other side.

LET'S TWIST

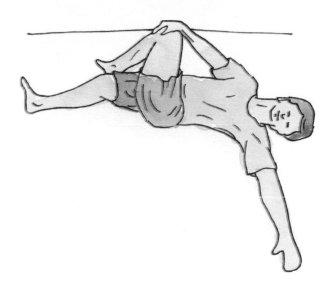

Start by lying on your back. Pull one knee to your chest and gently pull
the leg across your body with the opposite hand placed on the outside
of the knee. Extend the other arm out to the side at shoulder level. To

explore sensations in this shape, move your head side to side. Play with the angles of your flexed hip. Take notice for a few breath cycles.

When you feel ready, repeat on the other side. If you notice tension anywhere in your body, give yourself a pat on the back for recognizing this sensation, then soften, and let go. Also give yourself credit when you notice areas in your body that feel good.

WIDE WINDSHIELD WIPERS

Start by lying on your back, feet flat on the floor and slightly wider than hip-width apart. Your hands can be behind your head, at your side or on your belly. Find what works for you in the moment.

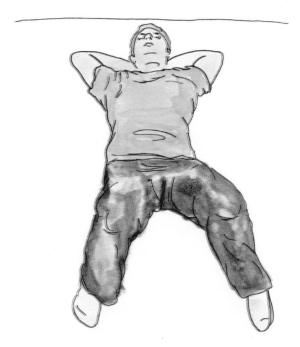

Then slowly and mindfully 'windshield-wipe' your knees to one side. Bring awareness to the different sensations you may feel comparing the right and left sides of your body. Pause for a few breaths here. Then slowly bring your knees back to the center. Now 'windshield-wipe' to the other side, again taking notice of how your body feels compared to the other side. No judgments. Just curious observations. Pause to connect with your breath here.

Suggestions for play include continuously rocking side to side, maintaining a slow and relaxed breathing pace. Notice the movement of your hips on your pelvis, the pelvis moving with your lower back, and even the rotation of your shoulders as you explore this movement. Try adding in some alternate arm raises as you move your lower body.

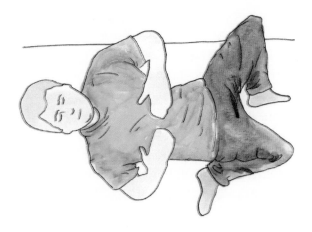

SUPPORTED BRIDGE

For this restorative pose, you can use pillows, bolsters, stacks of folded-up blankets, a squishy ball, or a yoga block. Explore with a variety of objects to notice the different sensations and pressures you feel and also to figure out what your preference is. Your nerve sensors are unique to you and have their own preferences as well.

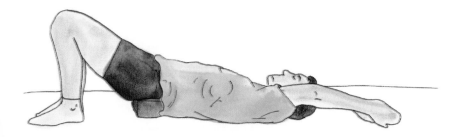

Once you find what works for you, allow your hips to melt down to rest on what you have placed below them. As you lie here in constructive rest, bring awareness to your breath. Where do you notice it most? Maybe you observe your breath in various parts of your body, like at the collarbone, chest, belly, or pelvic bowl. Notice these sensations change as your attention shifts to and from different areas.

To experience this in a more dynamic sense, remove the support from underneath you, allowing your back and hips to lie comfortably on the surface below. While gently pressing your feet into the ground, raise your hips towards the ceiling, visualize peeling your tailbone, hips, and lower back off the ground then slowly lower your hips back down.

Do this a few times, noticing the sensation of your hips as it articulates with your pelvis, the subtle movements of your vertebrae as you extend and flex your spine while moving up and down. Pay attention with purpose.

Once you gain an appreciation for this movement, synchronize your breath with the movement. It doesn't really matter if you breathe in or out. Life doesn't always balance perfectly on an inhale or an exhale. Variability and adaptability are what matters.

Add another layer of focus by raising your arms up above your head at the same time you raise your hips. See if you can elevate and land both movements at the same time. Most importantly, have fun!

KNEES TO CHEST

Begin lying on your back. On your next exhale, pull both your knees to your chest and give yourself a gentle squeeze (no death grip). Allow your shoulders to soften and melt down as you bring awareness to your natural breathing rhythm. Maybe you can feel your belly rise and fall against your thighs. Maybe you can feel the sensations of your pelvic muscles expand and gently recoil as you breathe in and out. Whatever you feel, take notice with curiosity. As you observe from a distance, you create space between you, your thoughts and your sensations.

It might feel good for you to explore moving in and out of this ball shape. Inhale into a starfish, extending legs and arms out in opposite

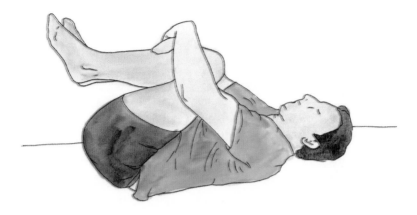

directions then exhale into a ball. Feel the differences between these two shapes as you transition in and out of each one.

PIGEON POSE

Start on all fours, in a table-top position. Rock your hips side to side, front and back. Feel the sensations of your pelvis articulating with your hips. Then, slide one knee in between your hands. The knee should be closer to one hand and the foot towards the other hand, with the outer edge of the lower leg resting on the ground.

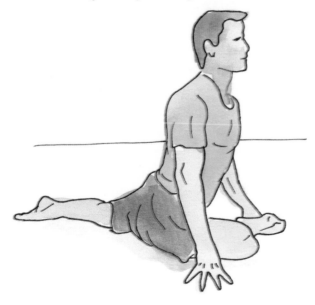

Next straighten your other leg, resting the top of the knee and foot on the floor. If this provides you with enough sensations, stay here. If you're looking for a bit more, lower yourself down onto your forearms. If you're feeling like the kinda guy who can bend himself into any shape, lower yourself all the way by sliding your arms out straight in front of you. Remember to breathe and soften your butt, hips and pelvic floor muscles.

Pause here to notice the change in pressure, stretch and intensity as you melt into this shape. Before moving on to the other side, take a moment to close your eyes and feel the differences in your entire body, not just the bits that hurt. (This goes for all the shapes you try!) Explore on the other side.

SEATED FORWARD BEND

Start by finding an easy seat on the floor, legs straight out in front of you. Adjust the comfort of your seat with blankets, blocks, pillows or a bolster. Experiment to see what is the most comfortable for you. Remember, we're pleasure-hunting here.

Slowly reach your hands forward, hinging at your hips with your back lengthened. You might begin to feel sensations in the back of your thighs and lower back as you sink deeper into this shape.

Don't fret if you can't reach your toes and don't push it either. Yes, it's okay to round your back as long as it feels good for you in your body. Just slide your hands as far down as comfortable and pause there for a few breaths. It could be as far as your thighs, below the knees, shins or

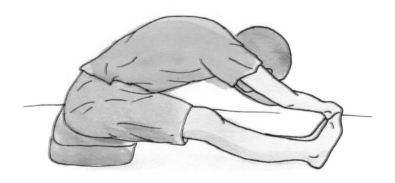

toes. Adjust as needed. A long strap could also be helpful here. If you're using a strap, sling it around the arches of your feet and use it as an anchor as you bend forward into the posture.

If comfortable, breathe consciously into your belly and the pelvis for several breaths. As you breathe in, notice a gentle expansion of your pelvic floor muscles and a widening of your sitz bones.

Another variation is to keep one knee bent with the sole of the foot touching the inner thigh of the extended leg. Or maybe you play with some counter pressure with the soles of your feet against a wall in front of you. Whatever you choose to do, don't forget to check in with yourself, observing what this is doing for your body and your mind (without judgment, of course).

STANDING FORWARD FOLD

Begin standing with your feet slightly wider than hip-width apart. Fold forward, visualizing each spinal segment rolling vertebrae by vertebrae.

Let yourself hang like a rag doll. Explore swaying your torso side to side, shaking your head no, then nodding your head yes. Play with your arm position. What does it feel like to cradle your elbows versus letting

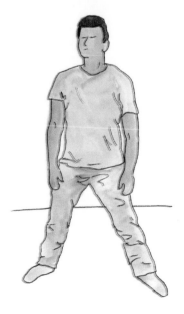

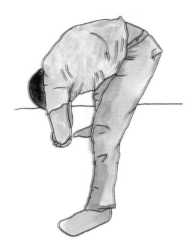

them hang to drape onto the floor? Maybe you find your yumminess holding onto your ankles. Take a few breaths to discover the sensations of your body here and really let yourself go. Feel free to investigate this posture with your legs closer together and wider apart. You've got choices.

Other suggestions you might want to consider is leaning into a wall behind you, or using a bolster or a few pillows on the floor to support your head.

STANDING BACKWARD BEND

Find a comfortable standing position and place your hands on your lower back. Take a moment to feel the sensations of your breath against your hands on your back. On your next breath out, extend your spine back as far as you feel is comfortable. Let your belly feel soft and the front of your neck be long. You can choose to keep your head neutral or extend to look up towards the ceiling. Again, see what this feels like for you as you dive into this shape. Investigate the sensations in your entire body as you move back and forth between standing neutral and bending backwards. Do you find yourself in the same position every time or do you notice yourself going a little further each time? How do the sensations change? If it feels good to stay in this posture for a few breath cycles, go for it.

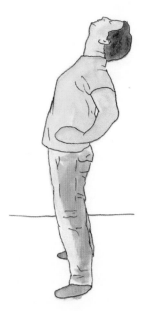

If you're itching for another variation, add in some arm movements. Here's one you can try on for size shown in the picture below.

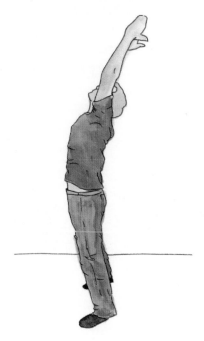

LOW LUNGE

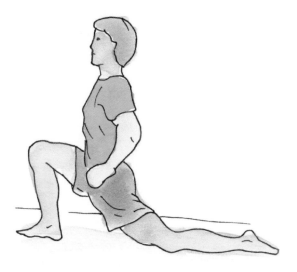

Start by kneeling on one leg with the other leg extended straight back, with the top of the foot resting on the floor.

Keeping your upper body relaxed and upright, lean forward, shifting your weight onto the front leg. Feel free to explore rocking back and forth into the stretch, and even doing some small hip circles in both directions. Maybe you challenge your balance and stretch your arms up towards the ceiling. Maybe it feels good to place your hands on top of your knee or palms on the floor. Check inwards to see how your body is feeling. After a few breaths, switch to do the other side, but before you do, pause to notice any differences you feel in your body comparing right and left side.

It might feel comfortable to have a blanket or pillow under the knee that is on the ground; if you don't need it, skip it.

INNER THIGH STRETCH

Find a step, curb, chair, pretty much anything you can confidently prop your leg on. Start with a small-to-medium step height or no step at all. The best part is you get to move around to figure out what you like. No

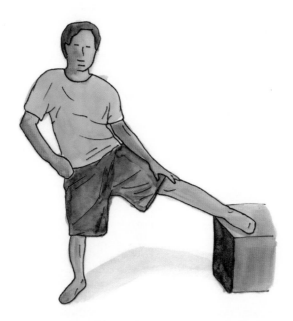

fixed rules! Place one leg onto the step, keeping the knee softly straight. Play with bending the knee on the standing leg to adjust the intensity of the sensation felt in your inner groin.

Visualize your spine lengthened as if there were someone pulling a puppet string attached to the top of your head. Allow your hips to face forward naturally or play with some movement.

Explore with what it feels like to move your pelvis around here. Maybe some tiny circles? Some side-to-side movements? Side bending your torso to and away from the leg propped up? How does this change the sensation you feel in your thigh, groin, back or pelvis? Again, just take note of sensations you might feel in other parts of your body.

Pause for a few breaths and switch to the other side, taking note of how your body feels after playing freely with this stretch.

THE SEE-SAW

Standing with your entire body facing front, bring one leg back behind you at a right angle so that the arch of your back foot lines up with the heel of your front foot that is pointing forward. Your feet will be perpendicular to each other. Let your pelvis adjust naturally to this

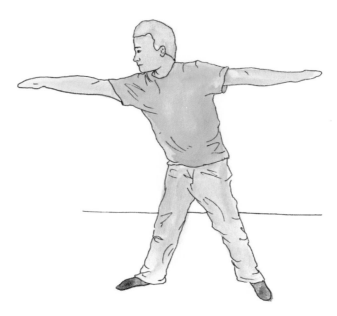

shape. How far apart your legs are from each other will depend on your comfort and preference. Having a wider stance might provide greater base of support and balance, greater range of movement and more sensations felt in the inner thighs. Maintain the front leg straight with toes pointed forward. Next, extend your arms out to a T at shoulder height, turn your head to look at the hand that is hovering over your front leg.

Now play with the top half of your body, shifting side to side. Feel the sensations of your rib cage as it floats back and forth over your pelvis. Feel the sides of your abdomen as you glide your torso over your pelvis. What sensations do you notice? This might feel nourishing for those nerves that come from your back, coursing through your abdomen and down into the pelvis and groin.

Then, lengthen the front arm forward as if you were reaching for something that was far from your reach. Side-bend your torso to lower your arm down to the inside of your knee, shin, ankle or foot. Explore what feels right for your body in the moment. There are a few options you can explore with your other hand: see what it feels like to put your hand on your hip, raise it up towards the ceiling, or place the back of your hand on the crest of your lower back. Try any or all of these and see how your sensations change with each one. You could turn your head to look down at your foot, straight ahead, or turn it to look up at your hand if your arm is raised up towards the ceiling.

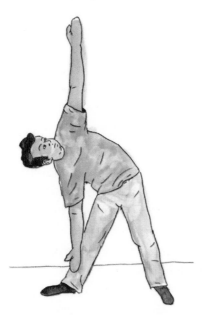

Again, feel free to move in and out of this posture, synchronizing this movement with your breath. Find your flow.

The purpose here is to use movement and postures to gain a new perspective of pain and to experience sensations in your body through a different lens. If you're use to plowing through life like a bull in a china shop, maybe it's time to reconsider your approach. Through movement snacks, breath and awareness, you can perhaps soften up a bit, ease into the process, rather than rebelling. Ask yourself: do I need to fight so hard?

PHYSICAL ACTIVITY, EXERCISE AND COUCH POTATO SYNDROME

In all likelihood, like many other men in similar scenarios, you've probably avoided your exercise routine for fear that it will make things worse. Maybe you're even thinking exercise is what got you into this mess in the first place or that you'll do more injury or harm to yourself that way.

Before we go any further, let's define physical activity and exercise. Physical activity is anything that encourages your body to kick into gear, exerting effort beyond your typical baseline. Sitting on the couch clicking your TV remote doesn't count as physical activity, sorry fellas. This is what we would call sedentary behavior. Exercise is physical activity that is intentionally scheduled, structured, and repetitive in nature with the goal of upping your health and fitness game. Both physical activity and exercise promote health and wellbeing. Whatever your feelings about physical activity and pain, know that exercise benefits far outweigh the risks of leading a physically inactive and sedentary lifestyle (cardiovascular disease, increased risk for all-cause mortality, cancer, declining muscle strength and function, inflammation, poor sleep, diabetes, obesity, and – you probably guessed it – a poorly functioning penis).[217] [218]

The aftermath of physical inactivity can have negative impacts on your pain, too. In ongoing pain situations, the likelihood of tissue injury or damage is slim, as average tissue healing times have long since passed.[219] Experiencing pain beyond this timeframe is mostly likely attributed to many complex processes involved in maintaining an ongoing state of protection. This is not to say that you should push through pain. Instead, it's to help boost your confidence that although tissues feel sensitive, you're safe to move (whether that's to help with the pain or mitigate the side effects of sedentary behavior).

So, we know that physical activity and exercise are good for us, but what exactly is happening under the hood that allows us to reap the rewards, especially analgesic effects? Proposed mechanisms include descending pain modulation (the brain's ability to dampen or amplify sensory messages) via specialized nerve receptors, decreasing excitability and sensitivity of the central nervous system, altering neuroimmune signaling in the CNS, and releasing your brain's own powerful painkilling drugs like dopamine, endogenous opioids and serotonin to assist with descending pain modulation.[220] [221] [222] Even short bouts of acute exercise have a positive influence on neuroplasticity, mood regulation, attention, focus, decision-making, stress, mental flexibility, tissue health, and so on.[223] Exercise also activates the HPA axis and can be used to work with anxiety-provoking feelings like heart rate increase, breath changes and motor output changes to help reframe these stress-response mechanisms into less of a threat when they occur during times of a flare-up or other fear-inducing situations.

Regular exercise, when done over a long period of time, has pain-relieving effects and decreases pain. This helps reorganize your nervous system pathways and immune system in such a way that switches from pain to analgesia.[224]

At the time of writing the second edition of this book, hot off the press, a few published studies are demonstrating that aerobic exercise can decrease bladder hypersensitivity, bladder pain, and urinary frequency in rats after a psychologically induced stressor (poor furry pals stood on a block surrounded with water, sorta like being stranded on an island). Researchers also noticed that exercise altered brain activity in areas that mediate the neurological peeing reflex. There was decreased brain activation to bladder-filling and positive neural integration with areas that influence the executive decision-making to inhibit or trigger the pee reflex. There's also speculation that the release of dopamine from exercise contributes to the brain-down dampening effect of nerve signals coming in from the body. In addition, exercise can modulate autonomic nervous system balance by increasing parasympathetic nervous system domination and soften the reins of the sympathetic nervous system.[225] [226]

Specific to men with CPPS and exercise, there is literature to support that adding an aerobic exercise regimen to your routine might be a great benefit in decreasing pain, anxiety, and urinary symptoms. Just as little as walking briskly for 40 minutes at 70-80% of your max heart rate three times a week might even do the trick.[227] According to the *Physical Activity Guidelines for Americans, 2nd edition*, health experts recommend 150 to 300 minutes of moderate intensity aerobic exercise per week (walking briskly) and two days devoted to building muscle (anything that makes your muscles work harder) for optimal health benefits.[228]

All this, while boosting your mood, quality of life and confidence, means you have something to do to help yourself, empowering you to take back control of your situation and life. These are recommendations not rules, so don't worry if this is more than you can chew right now. You'll still benefit from any activity (no matter how small) that gets you moving in the right direction and feeling better.

Physical activity and exercise have also been shown to have the potential to decrease the risk of getting CPPS in the first place.[229] Generally speaking, people who are more physically active tend to be more health-conscious and adopt healthier lifestyles and habits, though I'm well aware there are physically active people who aren't health conscious and that there are those who are physically active and health conscious who experience pelvic pain.

Bottom line: Exercise can change your physiological and psychological responses to pain, potentially lessening the severity of your pain, improving physical function, and positively influencing your psychological health and wellbeing, all of which can enhance your quality of life.[230]

Best yet, physical activity has no side effects other than potentially increasing muscle soreness, which goes away the more you do it, and possibly flare-ups, which means you need to pace yourself accordingly and build up your exercise tolerance gradually. As far as the intensity, frequency, and duration of exercise go, that's still up for debate. These parameters should be individually tailored to your needs and goals. And as always, consistency of any practice is important, so listen to your body and collaborate with your wellness team to find just the right amount of spice for your secret sauce.

More research is needed on the topic of exercise and the mechanisms by which it works on pain, as it's rather complex and there are many contributing factors that influence your pain experience. (Have I mentioned this yet? Oh yes, *ad nauseum.*) In general, it seems safe to say that you're better off moving. Even the slightest bit counts! The best exercise? Literature shows there isn't one. No specific exercise is better than another. In fact, all kinds of exercise can do the trick.[231] Something you actually *enjoy* doing and *will* do is the best kind of exercise for you.

CHAPTER 8

THE POWER OF TOUCH

Touch that is safe and pleasurable activates feel-good neurons and the release of chemicals in the brain that help calm down sensitivity and modulate pain response. The trick here is that you have to notice these feel-good moments, and your experience heavily depends on context. Context. Yup, it's so important that I'm mentioning it here, too.

Here comes another fun experiment for you to try. Close your eyes and think about the last time someone tickled you hard. What was your reaction? How did you feel? Hopefully, you didn't reflexively flail and punch the person. Now, with that fresh in your mind, go ahead and tickle yourself. Seriously, try to tickle yourself from every possible angle. Were you able to tickle yourself? Let me guess, you didn't have the same experience. Context means everything to your brain. A tickle is not a tickle unless someone else is doing the tickling. Touch is an experience that is highly dependent on who's doing the touching and whether you feel safe, confident and in control of any given situation.

SAFE TOUCH

The purpose of safe touch is to change the brain's interpretation of the parts that hurt, to minimize the need for protection, and to enhance your brain's ability to dampen incoming 'danger messages' from the body. In other words, we're de-threatening the situation (sorta like disarming a bomb).

In my opinion, treatment techniques shouldn't be painful. We don't treat pain with more pain. This is good because it means you don't have to endure deleterious modalities like injections, dry needling in your undercarriage, trigger point release devices, sitting on hard lacrosse balls, and for some, even a finger in the bum. There are other innocuous ways to work with the nervous system that don't include a dent in your wallet or you cringing just for the sake of so-called *recovery*.

Your spinal cord (the oldest part of your central nervous system) is a protector as well and has been designed to be sensitive to any potentially harmful stimuli. It will always try to be the boss, even without the brain or guts involved. To prove my point, take a second to look up 'dead fish alive' on YouTube (https://youtu.be/AWB3aOX_h4Y). The woman in the video is trying to scale the fish, without a head or guts, and finds herself 'fighting' him! This is a perfect example of the spinal cord and the withdrawal reflex.

All organisms have this innate protective mechanism, including you. This withdrawal reflex is responsive to sensory input, but it can also respond to your beliefs and thoughts, especially through anticipatory worry. Remember the story about Mike, the BB gun and his bruised balls? Your body may have flinched or tensed up just reading about that story. And I'm sure that's not the only time a thought has elicited this protective reflex.

According to physiotherapist Diane Jacobs, "The more the spinal cord tries to be protective by deploying its withdrawal reflex, the worse the situation may become for peripheral nerves: The last thing they (or any of their attached vessels) need is yet more compression or tensioning."[232] Sensory neurons are constantly firing and sending information up to your brain (the control center). Your brain's job is to filter out what's important and relevant from what's not. In the case of pain felt in your genital area, you can see how this information would not want to be ignored by your brain. These bits are important!

To take this one step further, some might say that the kind of touch applied to the tissues is not as important as the context or environment in which it is delivered. The associations made with any activity have great influence over your perception of that experience. Researchers have studied this in mice. Take a mouse from its comfy, safe, and familiar home, put it in another unfamiliar environment, and give it a shock there, the mouse will have elevated stress response biomarkers even 24 hours later. Now, take the same mouse, put it back in their comfy home, administer a shock there. These same biomarkers do not elevate, meaning it's not so much the shock itself that is the driver for these physiological changes, but the association with the environment in which the shock was delivered.[233]

Based on this, why would we want to activate this protective reflex even more with treatments that hurt? I hope you're convinced by now that the goal with manual therapy is to normalize your nervous system and immune responses to touch versus strengthening your threat detection systems.

HOW DOES MANUAL THERAPY WORK?

Like many of the other concepts you've already read, explaining 'how something works' isn't black and white. For the purposes of this book, I'm going to oversimplify the biologically plausible evidence for the reasons behind how non-painful manual therapy can help to reorganize the nervous system and provide analgesia.

In short, touch (and indeed, exercise) stimulate a different type of nerve fiber (a mechanoreceptor that senses change in pressure and stretch). This distracts the nerve fibers responsible for sending 'danger messages' to the brain.[234] [235] Whenever someone touches your skin, they are communicating with your nervous system and altering the input to your brain. Other mechanisms that might be playing into the mix include:

- ➤ Placebo
- ➤ Context (always a factor for the brain)
- ➤ Neurophysiological effects
- ➤ Local tissue effects (neurochemicals from nerve endings, immune cells, and changes in blood flow)
- ➤ All of the above.

This brings me to dispel some myths around fascia and trigger point therapy. For some of you, this could be a real jaw-dropper, so make sure to have a towel nearby to clean the drool off the floor.

MYOFASCIAL 'RELEASE'

Fascia is what connects everything in the body. It's kinda like cellophane wrapping around organs, muscles, bones, ligaments, tendons, blood vessels, and nerves. You name it, if it's in the body, it's got fascia. Fascia has nerve sensors that feed information to the brain. Fascia use to be thought of as not really having an important role. Today, there's more research to support that fascia does in fact play a part in posture and body movement. Fascia is an interconnected 3D webbing throughout the whole body that provides structural support and adaptability, disperses energy, and functions to allow for efficient and fluid movement.

So, if connective tissue is important for structural integrity, why would we want to change that? To put it bluntly, myofascial release is a bit of a misnomer because we're not releasing or 'stretching out' anything per se. There's no research that proves this really happens.[236][237][238] Just like muscle stretching, changes in range of motion or stiffness are most likely due to neurophysiological responses and molecular composition changes, rather than actual deformation of tissues. Although local tissue effects are also seen, like changes in blood flow, there is substantial evidence to prove this is not the *only* factor contributing to the changes you feel in your body. Tissues respond to mechanical and chemical input, and will adapt accordingly over time.

There is evidence to support both sides of the argument regarding what actually happens to connective tissues with movement, foam rolling, and fascial techniques.[239] Most likely it's a combination of local, global, neurophysiological, immune and contextual effects at play here. And let's not forget your belief and faith in the treatment, as well as the act of taking action to help yourself. (The brain calms down because you're doing something to take care of the issue.) If you believe something is good for you and that it will help you, it will. In this case, placebo can be a wonderful thing! Even people with chronic back pain that were told they're getting a placebo pill reported feeling less pain, stress, anxiety, and disability.[240]

Just know that the magic isn't in a special stretch, tool, or in someone's hands. It's all within you. *You* have the power to change your

The Power Of Touch

situation. You might just need a little nudge in the right direction to make that happen.

Don't get me wrong here. There are tissue changes that can occur due to misuse, disuse, inflammation, injury, stress, and so on, which is why all tissues need movement, blood flow and space for optimal health, as mentioned in the last chapter on movement. However, this is not the sole reason or blame for the experience of pain. To reiterate, muscle tone is highly influenced by the central nervous system, and anything that influences the nervous system will influence muscle tension. That includes any manual therapy, exercise, visual imagery, breathing, environment, thoughts, beliefs, what you're told, context, etc. So, I'm not saying that using hands, balls, foam rollers, rolling sticks, and other doohickeys don't play a role in therapy. These tools can be helpful to desensitize tender areas and get tissues feeling more normal again by applying certain pressures, friction, temperature, stretch, and other varying loads. You're using manual therapy to help your own body produce and release potent painkillers, increase blood flow and movement of tissues. In addition, you're hopefully providing some novel and soothing messages to your brain.

The key when applying any of these tools is to make sure that they feel yummy and allow you to feel safer in your body so that you can do things you enjoy with less pain. These modalities should encourage you to be more independent and empower you to do things for yourself, instead of being entirely dependent on them.

MYOFASCIAL TRIGGER POINTS: WHAT, WHY AND HOW

Myofascial trigger points are a popular yet controversial topic these days, not to mention the clever marketing around 'treating them,' which is a real money-maker. Some research argues that they exist while others dispute their existence.

Myofascial trigger points are a clinical phenomenon originally coined by Drs. Janet Travell and David Simons. It's thought that trigger points are fibrotic adhesions (nodules) within a taut band of muscle that

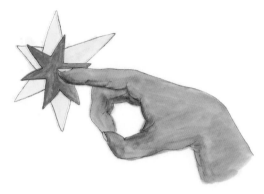

contribute to inflammation and sensitize nociceptors, which makes tissues hyper-irritable. All this rides on the premise that trigger points are an actual tissue pathology resulting from dehydration, overuse, repetitive strain, or injury.[241] [242] [243]

The actual definition of a trigger point is unclear across the literature (basically, no one can agree on what trigger points are). Diagnosing them is even more ambiguous as there is no universally accepted way of evaluating them, making examination highly unreliable. Indeed, scientists are having a hard time proving their existence. At most, studies have shown that individuals may feel differences in tissue with touch but nothing more. That said, even if they did exist, does this mean it's a pathology? The jury is leaning towards most likely not. Another reason being that these 'nodules' can be felt in some individuals who are not in pain.

Do we really need to make trigger points a thing at all then? In my opinion and that of many other scientists, the answer is probably not.

So, let me spare you some change. There's strong evidence that shows trigger points or muscle 'knots' don't exist and treating them seems to be a waste of resources.[244] [245] [246] [247] A cream of the crop research paper done by Denneny and colleagues made a bold statement to put the argument about the existence of trigger points to rest. "We do not recommend the use of TPMT [trigger point manual therapy] as a stand-alone treatment of chronic noncancer pain."[248] Interesting to note, in this same review, there were a few studies highlighted that reported pain worsening, specifically noted with internal pelvic manual therapy. The authors think that anxiety over the treatment may have contributed to the increase in pain reported.[249] The authors did not recommend more research be done on trigger point manual therapy as the collective evidence was so strong against using this treatment modality. In other words, they found no benefits. A different study revealed biochemical changes in 'active' trigger point tissue samples of symptomatic people, but that similar changes were also found in different muscle tissue samples that were not painful within the same individuals. This was said to indicate that the biochemical changes of tissues are not confined to the tissues that hurt, but that there might be more global effects of the central nervous and immune systems at play here.[250] [251] Even physical examination to find and diagnose trigger points is unreliable, and findings vary greatly between clinicians. Assessment also varies greatly, even with the same clinician repeating the testing on the same individuals.[252]

There are better plausible explanations based on the neurobiology of nociception and pain for having these hotspots. Perhaps trigger points amount to an altered state of neuroimmune function, altered central pain mechanisms, sensitized peripheral nerves, or when nerves release chemicals, making them backfire on themselves.[253] [254] [255] Basically, we know that there are tender spots that hurt. If we poke hard enough, we can make any tissue hurt. Go ahead and firmly squeeze your upper trap right now. Is it sensitive? I'm guessing, if you squeezed hard enough, it probably was!

What's the point of telling you all this? My hope is that you'll stop chasing a pipe dream! I kid, but in all seriousness, many manual therapy treatments are geared at treating myofascial pain and getting rid of trigger points, which only makes you think and believe that you have something structurally wrong with your body. It puts the blame on your muscles for all your troubles. I'm not denying that tender points exist, but there are better reasons for why tissues hurt than so-called muscle knots. The good news is that you don't have to endure and pay lots of money for someone to destroy them, going back to the reasoning that we don't treat pain with more pain. In fact, you can be gentle with yourself; no need to play whack-a-mole with these fictitious pathologies on your body.

Instead, here's what I suggest. Apply sensory techniques that help you reconnect with pleasure and joy in your body. Provide soothing sensory input to help your nervous system chill out. The same goes for anyone touching you. Seek pleasure not pain, because these both ride similar neurological pathways, but the goal is to reinforce the former. You should know that manual therapy is not the only tool you can use for your recovery; indeed, nor should it be. People get better no matter what we do.[256] In a nutshell, "on appraisal of the available scientific evidence, we would expect powerful safety cues that are delivered alongside the manual therapy are likely to be more potent analgesic triggers."[257] Although manual therapy might be better than doing nothing at all, this treatment alone might not offer lasting benefits in return.[258] [259] And just like exercise, there is no one superior manual therapy technique that is better than the rest.[260] [261] This is great news because specificity doesn't really matter, and you can keep things simple with regards to touch. Try novel things that are fun, tap into your curiosity, and most importantly, get back doing what you love.

Let's get hands-on with some sensory integration practice! Let me preface this by saying that there's no one single way to pleasure-hunt. You're going to have to try these suggestions out and experience them for yourself. Then modify or completely change them based on your own blueprint.

The goal with this activity is for you to start mapping out areas of safe touch and pleasure, create more positive experiences with touch resulting in less protection and eventually less pain.

Here are the basic principles of applying sensory integration:

> ➤ Do it several times a day to change the sensory input of what you feel in your body.
> ➤ Be intentional about it. In other words, pay attention to feeling good.
> ➤ Whatever you do should feel good or at least less crappy than it did before you started.
> ➤ Explore solo or with someone you feel safe and comfortable with.
> ➤ Keep it short and sweet as long as you pay attention.

You've already gotten some good practice with sensory integration earlier on. In this section specifically, we're going to explore safe touch.

TOUCHING WITH TOOLS

Using a variety of tools allows you to introduce novel sensory experiences for your nervous system. Tools can vary from using your hands to massage balls to anything that gives you the feel-goods. These next few hands-on strategies focus on areas around the pelvis. They may be helpful in desensitizing tender areas anywhere around your abdomen or above your pubic bone (area around the bladder). This may also be a good starting point if direct touch to your genitals is way too sensitive right now. Remember, that there is lots of crosstalk in these areas so safe and feel-good touch anywhere near the bits that hurt will help turn down the volume of sensitivity.

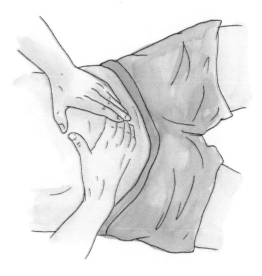

With your hands, explore the entire abdominal area from the bottom of your breast bone, lower ribs, down to your pubic bone. No need to be poky. Remember, we're pleasure-hunting not pain-hunting. Perhaps you just apply a static light touch to your belly and use your breathing to move the tissues under your hand. Or maybe you move your hands in a more active way for a little belly massage. Stay curious as you get in touch with your pleasure zones. Because there are no rules and manual therapy doesn't have to be specific. You can choose to move the skin of your belly in all sorts of ways, side to side, up and down, maybe adding in a little twist, how about a combination of all three? Take note of what feels good for you, bring in some breath awareness, rinse and repeat.

Massage balls are another tool you can use to help tissues and your nervous system adapt to various tissue demands and sensory stimuli. Massage balls come in all shapes, sizes, densities and textures. Softer balls will feel different than firmer or textured balls. If you've never experimented with massage balls, opt for the lighter, softer, smoother types. Again, choose one that looks yummy, interesting and inviting. If the thought of using a textured ball makes your cringe, it's probably not a good starting point.

How you use massage balls can also vary. You can lie on them. You can sit on them. You can use them as massage tools with your hands. You can explore what they feel like on various parts of your body, too. Let your sensory taste buds go wild. Pick an area to explore that feels safe, good or at least less sensitive to start.

Lying with your abdomen on a massage ball propped up or lying flat will offer a different sensory experience. You can be still and just breathe into it, or you can roll on it. Feel free to wiggle your legs, pelvis, or torso. Just like with movement snacks, stay in touch with your sensory experience rather than the narrative. If an area feels too sensitive, find a different area to explore. Revisit the sensitive area to see if anything has changed afterwards.

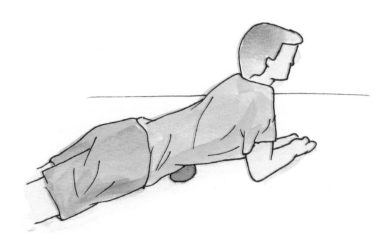

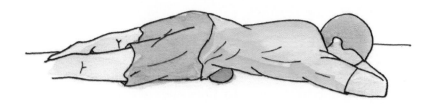

Lying with your back on the massage balls will also offer different sensory stimuli. Again, here you can explore what it feels like with the balls at your lower back, mid-back, upper back. Arms along your side or above your head, knees bent or straight. Add some movement if you'd like too, rolling up and down, side to side. Balls placed at your lower back might provide feedback for your breath sensations as you tune into the sensations of your breath at your lower back.

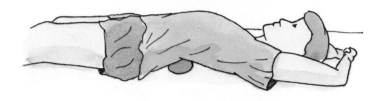

These were just a few ideas to get your creative juices flowing. There are many ways to tailor these types of strategies to your specific needs, so if you need more guidance, feel free to connect with me at drsusieg. com. Alternatively, you can consult with your wellness team.

DIRECT SENSORY INTEGRATION TO THE PERINEUM, SCROTUM AND/OR PENIS[262]

The idea here is to map out areas that feel good, less good, and not good. Like a stop light: green, yellow, red. Start applying gentle touch to areas on your body that you know are green light, then slowly work your way closer and closer to the areas that are more sensitive. The area that you touch first is the area that will be flooded the most with sensory input, so go slow and use breathing to help calm any nerves during the process. Remember, you're in charge of how much pressure, stretch, and touch you apply. The purpose is to provide persistent, purposeful touch to these areas to restore tolerance to touch and help tissues adapt to a diversity of touch like stretch, friction, sheer, pressure, etc.

You could gently massage the taint area or your penis. Or maybe you stretch the scrotum. Whatever you choose to do, work slowly with compassionate curiosity. Breathe and soften into the process without overanalyzing.

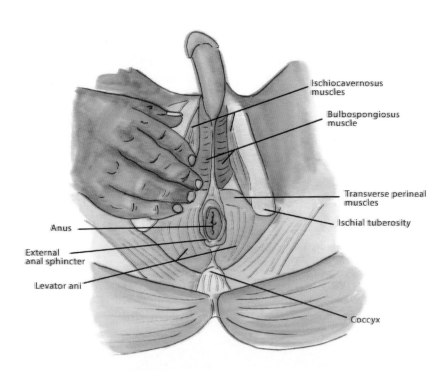

Pay attention to the quality of sensations you feel, like stretch, pressure, texture and temperature, rather than thinking in terms of good or bad, right or wrong. Drop the storyline and instead get absorbed in your sensory experience (cue *clean* pain versus *dirty* pain again).

It's unrealistic to expect that you're going to be feeling yourself up several times a day, so finding opportunities to provide purposeful, pleasurable touch will be key. Here are some potentials:

> In the shower while you're lathering up, feel the quality of sensations on your hand and on the rest of your body.
> While you're drying off, pay attention to the sensations of your favorite towel touching your skin.
> When masturbating (if that's a part of your lineup), feel the sensations of your hand on your penis. Play with varying pressure, shear, stretch and using lubricant. Lubrication is a novel texture that can change your experience and add some fun. The brain loves novelty!

You don't always have to be naked to reap the benefits of touch either. Proprioceptive folds are a great way to get sensory input of movement and touch into your day. Proprioception is your sensory awareness (internal radar) of movement and body position. Go ahead and close your eyes, raise your arm up in the air. Where is your arm? How do you know where it is?

Specialized mechanoreceptors in skin, muscles, joints and tendons, fascia, and pretty much all over the rest of your body detect changes in tissue movement and body position and feed this information to the boss, your brain, where it is further processed and integrated with many other sensory systems like vision, hearing, and balance for an overall representation of where your body is in space.[263] [264] As a result, you have a conscious experience of what your body is doing and what it feels like. All this is created by your brain based on the information provided.

Recall that your brain has dedicated body maps that help you sense and move your body parts. With persistent pain, we know these maps change and become less precise. Having an accurate and precise body map is essential to coordinated, fluid and non-painful movement. Confused maps can lead to distorted body images and sensations felt in the body. Phantom limb pain, which I mentioned earlier, is a perfect example of this distortion. The body part is gone, but the body map devoted to that part still exists, and a person can still experience pain in a body part that is no longer there.

The brain uses all sensory information to make sense of the world around you in any given context. It will often play tricks on you. Just take a look at this picture, what do you see?

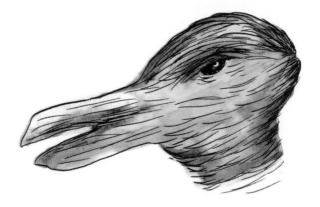

Let me just change the orientation of the same picture just a bit. Now what do you see?

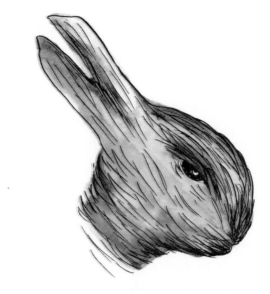

You probably saw a duck in the first picture and then a rabbit in the second. Same picture but two different experiences. Your brain won't allow you to see both at the same time, but it will wrangle the two, for sure… duck, rabbit, duck, rabbit, duck. Based on the orientation, your brain will choose the one that makes the most sense. If you need a refresher of the science behind this topic, go back and re-read Chapter 3.

Maps are refined, defined, and primed via visual imagery, touch and movement! Slow, purposeful, and safe touch and movement will help to train your brain to experience less pain. Avoiding movement, sitting, or sexual activity can have unhelpful effects on your recovery, so the goal is to build up positive experiences until you feel more and more confident with touch and activity, including sexual function.

Science review over, let's move on to proprioceptive folds. This exercise is one way you can refine your body maps, provide safe touch, and calm your nervous system.

Standing tall, place your hands on the crest of your lower back. As you breathe out, slide your hands down the front of your hips, thighs and lower legs and come into a forward fold. Then as you breathe in, slide your hands up from your feet to the hips and lower back as you come back up to standing. Transition slowly as if you were moving in a vat of honey. Notice sounds, textures, sensations in the hands, and how these sensations change as you move. Repeat this for a few breath cycles.

Next, try this activity again, but this time pay attention to the movement of your lower back moving on top of your pelvis, your pelvis moving on your hips, your thighs articulating with your knees and how your lower leg moves on top of the ankle. Then reverse the awareness as you explore on your way up. Maintain a natural and comfortable breathing pace. What do you notice?

There's no one single way to do sensory integration. It's more about reconnecting with your body in ways that hurt less and feel good.

WHERE DOES INTERNAL WORK FIT IN?

Let me start this section by making it plain: you don't have to do internal work to get better. I know that some male bodies out there are hesitant and find the thought of putting anything up their butt a bit intimidating. Not to mention the mainstream cultural taboos around this topic. If you're hesitant or anxious about internal work, know that you're not alone and definitely not doomed.

Pelvic therapy doesn't have to be all about internal work, either. You and your therapist should collaborate together on the best starting point for you. This relationship should be built on trust and partnership. Remember, feeling safe is an important part of your recovery. Internal work should be meaningful and match your individual goals and needs.

That being said, remember my rant about muscle tightness and tension? The same goes with your pelvic muscles. How do we measure pelvic tightness and relaxation? What is normal? There is really no way of accurately measuring this. Tightness and tension are subjective both by the person experiencing it and the clinician assessing. Context (umm, like a finger in the butt) will also change the motor response, bodily and mental reactions. I encourage you and your clinician to avoid language that would encourage fixation on structural tightness and instead shift towards just a general sense of body awareness of the pelvis and elsewhere. Remember, tension doesn't have to be scary.

Some people find using an internal tool like a wand or dilator helpful, so should you or shouldn't you give it a try? It depends… What would be the purpose of doing internal work for you? For example, did you use to enjoy anal play and now can't because of pain? Are bowel movements painful? In such cases, internal work might be an option to explore. There has to be a reason to do internal work that would make it purposeful for you. Just like direct sensory integration to the perineum, penis and scrotum, you can apply the same principles with internal therapy. The idea is to promote circulation to tissues, restore tolerance to normal touch, function, and movement.

If you're open-minded and willing to explore internal work (for whatever reason), there is no harm in doing so, but if you're really not interested, just pass. It's like someone telling you that you have to swim laps for exercise when you hate anything that has to do with being in the water. You either won't do it, or you'll do it ruefully.

Internal work can be done solo, with a partner or with a pelvic health clinician. There are many ways to address internal work that feel safe and comfortable. You can choose to use your own finger, a wand, a dilator, or any anal tool or toy of your choice based on your own preference and tissue tolerance. (You have permission to explore with toys or not depending if that is part of your sexual menu. The point is this internal work doesn't have to be clinical, but can be fun and pleasurable.)

If you've never experienced internal work, it would be best to have some guidance so that you can build confidence to do it on your own. Again, no rules other than not treating pain with more pain and making sure you're using safe touch to feel good. We're not chasing trigger points. Your job is the map out areas that feel good, less good, and not good, then reinforce what you enjoy and try to change what you don't.

Here is a suggested guideline for internal manual therapy:

1. Wash your hands.
2. Start by getting yourself comfortable. A suggestion: prop yourself up in bed and use plenty of pillows so your back is relaxed and supported.
3. You can bend your knees. A suggestion: use pillows to support outer knees so you don't have to stress holding them up.
4. Spend a few minutes taking some slow, soft breaths to settle in.
5. Apply generous amounts of lubricant to finger, wand, dilator, etc. Any lubricant of your choice will do. Note that silicone lubricant is not recommended for use with silicone tools or toys.
6. Gently lift your penis and testicles up and out of the way.
7. Find your anus. If you need help, use a mirror.
8. Orient yourself to the anal opening like a clock, 12 o'clock being your pubic bone (in front), and 6 o'clock, your anal opening (see image on page 182).
9. Gently, slowly insert the tip of your finger or tool of choice into the anal opening, which is at 6 o'clock. Take a few moments to breathe here. If there's some discomfort or difficulty with insertion, don't force it. Try to gently squeeze your pelvic floor muscles and let go. Do this a few times allowing your body to lead insertion versus you pushing in. You can progress with insertion as far as it is safe and comfortable to do so. (Depth of insertion may vary depending on your tool of choice).

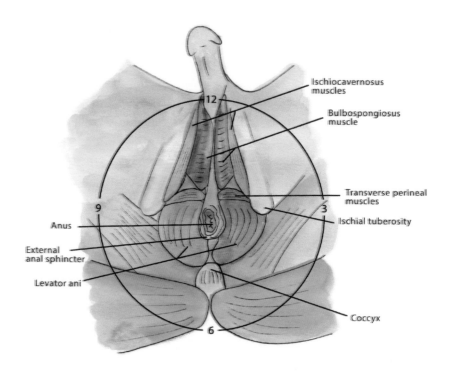

10. As you breathe in and out, feel the expansion and lengthening of your pelvic floor muscles. You might feel your anus opening and slightly expanding outward with every in-breath. You can do this for 1, 2,3 or 5 minutes – whatever feels right for you at that time.

11. Once you feel ready to move on, experiment with sensations as you gently tense and release your pelvic muscles. Vary the amount of tension. For example, what does it feel like when you squeeze 25%, 50%, 75%, 100%? What does it feel like when you let go? You can try letting go in the same incremental way, too.

12. If you feel comfortable to continue and things feel good, you can explore with different types of sensory touch like sweeping, shearing (moving in and out) and pressure. Using your finger or tool of choice, slowly begin to introduce in movement. Maybe you sweep from the pubic bone to the tail bone on one side, then the other. Maybe you shear in and out. Or maybe you add

progressive pressure to different areas within the pelvic bowl. Be mindful of the prostate nestled at 12'o'clock. Remember, go slow to let your nervous system adapt accordingly to the sensory input provided.

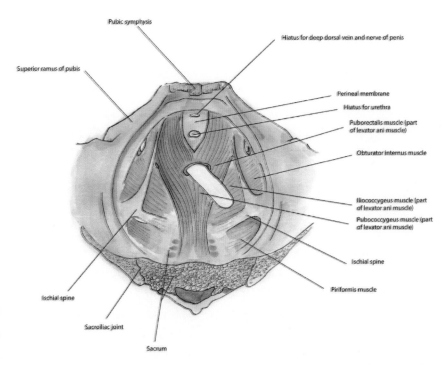

Always use caution when exploring new self-help techniques for the first time. If you're afraid or worried that you'll hurt yourself or make things worse, that defeats the purpose of down-regulating an overly sensitive nervous system. It's wise to consult with a pelvic health therapist for more guidance and support.

Again, the above suggestion is just a suggestion, and an individualized approach is always best.

CHAPTER 9

DON'T GIVE UP!

While there's so much more I'd love to write about and teach you, this is not a textbook. Your body is unique. Treating it doesn't stop here at the page. What I've shared with you will guide you in the right direction and give you support on your health journey. Who knows? Maybe you even had a good laugh here and there! (Humor me, please!)

Every person responds differently to what they try so I can't guarantee how you're going to feel, but if you trust in the process, everything else will fall into place. Sometimes fear is what blocks us from truly being free. So, the next time you think this is never going to go away, ask yourself: what if the opposite were true?

WHEN THE GOING GETS TOUGH, FIND THE RIGHT BUFFS

You may have heard of the African proverb: it takes a village to raise a child. Well, the same goes for persistent pelvic pain. It takes a team of wellness practitioners to support you throughout your recovery, so never feel like you have to go through this alone.

Wellness practitioners worth having by your side include:

- ➤ Sexual medicine physician
- ➤ Pelvic health therapist
- ➤ Urologist
- ➤ Gastroenterologist
- ➤ Health coach
- ➤ Massage therapist

- ➤ Yoga therapist
- ➤ Acupuncturist
- ➤ Nutritionist
- ➤ Psychologist or licensed clinical social worker
- ➤ Sex and relationship therapist
- ➤ Physiatrist specializing in pain

Of course, this isn't an exhaustive list, and you might not need all the people on this list. These are just some common providers that might be helpful along your journey. It's worth saying that we're not all created equal. Just because you had a so-so experience with one practitioner doesn't mean that the next one will be just like them. So, don't be afraid to get multiple opinions or consultations. Trust your intuition. Find the best team that suits your needs and, most importantly, that believes you, validates your experience, takes the time to listen, and collaborates with you. You bring your own unique strengths and resources to the table. No one is going to 'fix' you, because you're not broken. We are here to share our expertise, knowledge, and support, but ultimately, you're the expert in *you*.

YOU CAN LIVE A LIFE WITHOUT PAIN

Persistent pelvic pain takes courage, compassion, commitment and patience to tackle the good, the bad and the ugly that comes with it. This is a crockpot not a microwave kinda deal. You might not be able to stop pain from knocking at your door, but you certainly have the choice to not suffer. Don't let pain define your world. I'm sure there's a whole helluva lot more you'd like to be doing. So, get up, get moving, and keep on keepin' on.

That said, if you've read this far and practiced the techniques but need more guidance, don't be afraid to come find it! We all need to do some troubleshooting from time to time. Questions might arise… What am I supposed to be feeling? I put my hand where? What else can I do for…? Am I doing this right? These questions are common.

If you're anything like me, maybe you thrive with some one-on-one support and would like a coach to guide you through the process. That undivided attention is so helpful, which is why I created several health programs that help men with pelvic pain to become experts in treating themselves.

If you're ready to take matters into your own hands (no pun intended!) then connect with me at drsusieg.com to become the boss of your own health.

In loving wellness for your pelvis,

Dr. Susie Gronski, PT, DPT

ABOUT THE AUTHOR

Specializing in men's pelvic and sexual health, **Susie Gronski, PT, DPT**
is a licensed doctor of physical therapy, certified pelvic rehabilitation
practitioner, international teacher
and creator of one-to-one and self-
paced health programs that help
men with pelvic pain become experts in treating themselves.

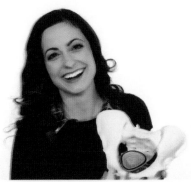

Her passion is making you feel
comfortable about taboo subjects like sex and private parts. Social
stigmas aren't her thing and neither is medical fluff. She provides real
advice, just like a friend who knows the lowdown down below. She's
determined to make sure you know you can get help for:

➤ painful ejaculation
➤ problems with the joystick
➤ discomfort or pain during sex
➤ controlling your pee

Without being embarrassed… So, if you're having some trouble
'down there', she's the person to get to know. Learn more by visiting
drsusieg.com.

GLOSSARY

For ease of reference, here are some definitions of the common terms used in this book.

Term	Definition
allostatic load	cumulative burden on your bodily systems and mind
autonomic	bodily systems functioning involuntarily and automatically
autonomic nervous system	consisting of the parasympathetic, sympathetic, and enteric nervous systems that regulate involuntary bodily functions like heart rate and digestion
central nervous system	system controlling most functions of the body, comprising the brain and spinal cord
descending pain modulation	brain and spinal cord ability to dampen or amplify incoming sensory messages from the body

distributed process	process happening across several interrelated and interconnected areas
enteric nervous system	division of the autonomic nervous system relating to the gut
homeostasis	balance of bodily processes
insular cortex	region of the brain involved with sensory and motor processing, sense of internal wellbeing, emotions, consciousness, learning, and other brain functions
ischial tuberosities	bones of the pelvis that you sit on (also called *sitz bones*)
microbiome	ecosystem of microorganisms that live on and inside of the body
micturition	entire process of urination (peeing)
neural circuits	collection of neurons that connect together to carry out a specific function
neuro	related to the nervous system
neurohormones	hormones that act like chemical messengers released

	from specialized nerve cells in the brain, adrenal glands, and gut
neurotags	collection of nerve cells and immune cells in the brain that activate across multiple areas of the brain in a particular pattern to produce an output
nociception	multidimensional process triggered by 'danger sensors' that the brain processes to consider the overall emotional and biological importance of the sensory signal
parasympathetic nervous system	'rest and digest' response system
physiological	related to bodily functions of living organisms, anything that has to do with the body and its normal functions
proprioception	sensory awareness of body position and movement
sympathetic nervous system	'fight, flight, or freeze' response system
upregulated	increased response to stimulus
wand	tool or toy for internal work

REFERENCES

Don't worry, I didn't make this up. I stand on the shoulders of giants, the pioneers, clinicians, researchers, educators, and most importantly the heroes who came through their journey with pain, all of whom have sacrificed their blood, sweat and tears to pave the way for pain science in order to revolutionize pain care and lessen suffering for those who hurt. But if you want to nerd out and read some dry, medical journal articles, then knock yourself out. Below are the references. Happy reading!

(Endnotes)

1   Collins, M. M., Stafford, R. S., O'Leary, M. P., & Barry, M. J. (1998). How common is prostatitis? A national survey of physician visits. *The Journal of Urology, 154*(4), 1224-1228.

2   Darnall, B. D., Scheman, J., Davin, S., Burns, J. W., Murphy, J. L., Wilson, A. C., Kerns., R. D., & Mackey, S. C. (2016). Pain psychology: A global needs assessment and national call to action. *Pain Medicine, 17*(2), 250-263. doi:10.1093/pm/pnv095

3   Anothaisintawee, T., Attia, J., Nickel, J. C., Thammakraisorn, S., Numthavaj, P., McEvoy, M., & Thakkinstian, A. (2011). Management of chronic prostatitis/chronic pelvic pain syndrome. *JAMA, 305*(1), 78-86. doi:10.1001/jama.2010.1913

4   Loeser, J. D., Arendt-Nielsen, L., Baron, R., Basbaum, A., Bond, M., Breivik, H., & et al. (2011). Classification of chronic pain: Descriptions of chronic pain syndromes and definitions of pain terms. In (2nd ed.). Seattle: IASP Press. Retrieved from https://www.iasp-pain.org/PublicationsNews/Content.aspx?ItemNumber=1673

5   Collins, M. M., Stafford, R. S., O'Leary, M. P., & Barry, M. J. (1998). How common is prostatitis? A national survey of physician visits. *The Journal of Urology, 154*(4), 1224-1228.

6   Doiron, R., Shoskes, D., & Nickel, J. C. (2019). Male CP/CPPS: Where do we stand? *World Journal of Urology, 37*, 1015-1022. doi:10.1007/s00345-019-02718-6

7   Magistro, G., Wagenlehner, F., Grabe, M., Weidner, W., Stief, C., & Nickel, J. C. (2016). Contemporary management of chronic prostatitis/chronic pelvic pain syndrome. *European Urology, 69*(2), 286-297. doi:10.1016/j.eururo.2015.08.061

8   Krieger, J. N., Nyberg, L., & Nickel, J. C. (1999). NIH consensus definition and classification of prostatitis. *JAMA, 282*(3), 236–237. doi:10-1001/pubs.JAMA-ISSN-0098-7484-282-3-jac90006

References

9   Krieger, J. N., Nyberg, L., & Nickel, J. C. (1999). NIH consensus definition and classification of prostatitis. *JAMA, 282*(3), 236–237. doi:10-1001/pubs.JAMA-ISSN-0098-7484-282-3-jac90006

10   Anothaisintawee, T., Attia, J., Nickel, J. C., Thammakraisorn, S., Numthavaj, P., McEvoy, M., & Thakkinstian, A. (2011). Management of chronic prostatitis/chronic pelvic pain syndrome. *JAMA, 305*(1), 78-86. doi:10.1001/jama.2010.1913

11   Doiron, R., Shoskes, D., & Nickel, J. C. (2019). Male CP/CPPS: Where do we stand? *World Journal of Urology, 37*, 1015-1022. doi:10.1007/s00345-019-02718-6-6

12   Collins, M. M., Meigs, J. B., Barry, M. J., Walker Corkery, E., Giovannucci, E., & Kawachi, I. (2002). Prevalence and correlates of prostatitis in the health professionals follow-up study cohort. *The Journal of Urology, 167*(3), 1363–1366.

13   Dewitt-Foy, M. E., Nickel, J. C., & Shoskes, D. (2019). Management of chronic prostatitis/chronic pelvic pain syndrome. *European Urology Focus, 5*, 2-4. doi:10.1016/j.euf.2018.08.027

14   Nickel, J. C., Alexander, R. B., Schaeffer, A. J., Landis, J. R., Knauss, J. S., Propert, K. J., & Chronic Prostatitis Collaborative Research Network Study Group. (2003). Leukocytes and bacteria in men with chronic prostatitis/chronic pelvic pain syndrome compared to asymptomatic controls. *The Journal of Urology, 170*(3), 818–822. doi:10.1097/01.ju.0000082252.49374.e9

15   Bowen, D. K., Dielubanza, E., & Schaeffer, A. J. (2015). Chronic bacterial prostatitis and chronic pelvic pain syndrome. *BMJ Clinical Evidence, 2015*(1802), 1-30.

16   Rees, J., Abrahams, M., Doble, A., & Cooper, A. (2015). Diagnosis and treatment of chronic bacterial prostatitis and chronic prostatitis/chronic pelvic pain syndrome: a consensus guideline. *BJU International, 116*(4), 509-525. doi:10.1111/bju.13101

17   Marchant, J. (2018). When Antibiotics Turn Toxic. *Nature, 555*, 431-433. doi:10.1038/d41586-018-03267-5

18   Doiron, R., & Nickel, J. C. (2018). Management of chronic prostatitis/chronic pelvic pain syndrome. *Canadian Urological Association Journal, 12*(6S3), S161-3. doi:10.5489/cuaj.5325

19   Nickel, J. C., Shoskes D., Wang, Y., Alexander, R. B., Fowler, J. E., Zeitlin S., O'Leary, M. P., Pontari, M. A., Schaeffer, A. J., Landis, R., Nyberg, L., Kusek, J. W., Propert, K. J., and the Chronic Prostatitis Collaborative Research Network Study Group. (2006). How does the pre-massage and post-massage 2-glass test compare to the Meares-Stamey 4-glass test in men with chronic prostatitis/chronic pelvic pain syndrome? *The Journal of Urology, 176*(1), 119-124. doi:10.1016/S0022-5347(06)00498-8.

20   Nickel, J. C., Stephens, A., Landis, J. R., Chen, J., Mullins, C., van Bokhoven, A., Lucia, M. S., Melton-Kreft, R., Ehrlich, G. D., & MAPP Research Network. (2015). Search for microorganisms in men with urologic chronic pelvic pain syndrome: A culture-independent analysis in the MAPP Research Network. *The Journal of Urology, 194*(1), 127–135. doi:10.1016/j.juro.2015.01.037

21   Schaeffer, A. J., Landis, J. R., Knauss, J. S., Propert, K. J., Alexander, R. B., Litwin, M. S., Nickel, J. C., O'Leary, M. P., Nadler, R. B., Pontari, M. A., Shoskes, D. A., Zeitlin, S. I., Fowler, J. E. Jr., Mazurick, C. A., Kishel, L., Kusek, J. W., Nyberg, L. M., & Chronic Prostatitis Collaborative Research Network Group. (2002). Demographic and clinical characteristics of men with chronic prostatitis: the national institutes of health chronic prostatitis cohort study. *The Journal of Urology, 168*(2), 593–598.

References

22   Schaeffer, A. J., Landis, J. R., Knauss, J. S., Propert, K. J., Alexander, R. B., Litwin, M. S., Nickel, J. C., O'Leary, M. P., Nadler, R. B., Pontari, M. A., Shoskes, D. A., Zeitlin, S. I., Fowler, J. E. Jr., Mazurick, C. A., Kishel, L., Kusek, J. W., Nyberg, L. M., & Chronic Prostatitis Collaborative Research Network Group. (2002). Demographic and clinical characteristics of men with chronic prostatitis: the national institutes of health chronic prostatitis cohort study. *The Journal of Urology, 168*(2), 593–598.

23   Astill, T., Cavaleri, R., & Chalmers, K. J. (2019). The impact of chronic pelvic pain in men: A new assessment tool. (Unpublished honours thesis at Western Sydney University, Sydney, Australia.)

24   Origoni, M., Leone Roberti Maggiore, U., Salvatore, S., & Candiani, M. (2014). Neurobiological mechanisms of pelvic pain. *Biomed Research International, 2014,* 1-9. doi:10.1155/2014/903848

25   Nickel, J. C., Tripp, D. A., Chuai, S., Litwin, M. S., McNaughton-Collins, M., Landis, J. R., Alexander, R. B., Schaeffer, A. J., O'Leary, M. P., Pontari, M. A., White, P., Mullins, C., Nyberg, L., Kusek, J., & NIH-CPCRN Study Group. (2008). Psychosocial variables affect the quality of life of men diagnosed with chronic prostatitis/chronic pelvic pain syndrome. *BJU International, 101*(1), 59–64. doi:10.1111/j.1464-410X.2007.07196.x

26   Chung, S., & Lin, H. (2013). Association between chronic prostatitis/chronic pelvic pain syndrome and anxiety disorder: a population-based study. *PLOS ONE, 8*(5), e64630. doi:10.1371/journal.pone.0064630

27   Tripp, D. A., Nickel, J. C., Wang, Y., Alexander, R. B., Propert, K. J., Schaeffer, A. J., Landis, R., O'Leary, M. P., Pontari, M. A., McNaughton-Collins, M., Shoskes, D. A., Comiter, C. V., Datta, N. S., Fowler, J. E., Nadler, R. B., Zeitlin, S. I., Knauss, J. S., Nyberg, L. M., Litwin, M. S., & Chronic Prostatitis Collaborative Research Network Study Group. (2006). Catastrophizing and pain-contingent rest predict patient adjustment in men with chronic prostatitis/chronic pelvic pain syndrome. *The Journal of Pain, 7*(10), 697-708. doi: 10.1016/j.jpain.2006.03.006

28   Riegel, B., Bruenahl, C. A., Ahyai, S., Bingel, U., Fisch, M., & Lowe, B. (2014). Assessing psychological factors, social aspects and psychiatric co-morbidity associated with chronic prostatitis/chronic pelvic pain syndrome in men—a systematic review. *Journal of Psychosomatic Research, 77,* 333-350. doi:10.1016/j.jpsychores.2014.09.012

29   Smith, K., Pukall, C., Tripp, D., & Nickel, J. C. (2006). Sexual and relationship functioning in men with chronic prostatitis/chronic pelvic pain syndrome and their partners. *Archives of Sexual Behavior, 36*(2), 301-311. doi:10.1007/s10508-006-9086-7

30   Rizzolatti, G., & Sinigaglia, C. (2016). The mirror mechanism: a basic principle of brain function. *Nature Reviews Neuroscience, 17*(12), 757-765. doi:10.1038/nrn.2016.135

31   Klein, H. (1991). Couvade Syndrome: Male counterpart to pregnancy. *The International Journal of Psychiatry in Medicine, 21*(1), 57-69. doi:10.2190/FLE0-92JM-C4CN-J83T

32   Moseley, L., & Butler, D. (2017). *Explain pain supercharged.* Noigroup Publications.

33   Cohen, D., Gonzalez, J., & Goldstein, I. (2016). The role of pelvic floor muscles in male sexual dysfunction and pelvic pain. *Sexual Medicine Reviews, 4*(1), 53-62. doi:10.1016/j.sxmr.2015.10.001

34   Astill, T., Cavaleri, R., & Chalmers, K. J. (2019). The impact of chronic pelvic pain in men: A new assessment tool. (Unpublished honours thesis at Western Sydney University, Sydney, Australia.)

References

35   Collins, M. M., Meigs, J. B., Barry, M. J., Walker Corkery, E., Giovannucci, E., & Kawachi, I. (2002). Prevalence and correlates of prostatitis in the health professionals follow-up study cohort. *The Journal of Urology, 167*(3), 1363–1366.

36   Anothaisintawee, T., Attia, J., Nickel, J. C., Thammakraisorn, S., Numthavaj, P., McEvoy, M., & Thakkinstian, A. (2011). Management of chronic prostatitis/ chronic pelvic pain syndrome. *JAMA, 305*(1), 78-86. doi:10.1001/jama.2010.1913

37   Bajic, P., Dornbier, R. A., Doshi, C. P., Wolfe, A. J., Farooq, A. V., & Bresler, L. (2019). Implications of the genitourinary microbiota in prostatic disease. *Current Urology Reports, 20*(34), 1-10. doi:10.1007/s11934-019-0904-6

38   Antunes-Lopes, T., Vale, L., Coelho, A. M., Silva, C., Rieken, M., Geavlete, B., Rashid, T., Rahnama'i., S. M., Cornu, J. N., Marcelissen, T., & EAU Young Academic Urologists Functional Urology Working Group. (2018). The role of urinary microbiota in lower urinary tract dysfunction: A systematic review. *European Urology Focus, 6*(2), 361-369. doi:10.1016/j.euf.2018.09.011

39   Cohen, D., Gonzalez, J., & Goldstein, I. (2016). The role of pelvic floor muscles in male sexual dysfunction and pelvic pain. *Sexual Medicine Reviews, 4*(1), 53-62. doi:10.1016/j.sxmr.2015.10.001

40   Dunbar, R. I. M., Baron, R., Frangou, A., Pearce, E., van Leeuwen, E. C. J., & Stow, J., Partridge, G., MacDonald, I., Barra, V., & van Vugt, M. (2011). Social laughter is correlated with an elevated pain threshold. *Proceedings of the Royal Society Biological Sciences, 279*(1731), 1161-1167. doi:10.1098/rspb.2011.1373

41   Cohen, D., Gonzalez, J., & Goldstein, I. (2016). The role of pelvic floor muscles in male sexual dysfunction and pelvic pain. *Sexual Medicine Reviews, 4*(1), 53-62. doi:10.1016/j.sxmr.2015.10.001

42   Jacobs, D. (2016). *Dermoneuromodulating: Manual treatment for peripheral nerves and especially cutaneous nerves.* Tellwell.

43   DeLancey, J., Jünemann, K., Thüroff, J., Dixon, J., Gosling, J., & Norton, P. (1994). Anatomy and function of the pelvic floor. In B Schussler, J Laycock, & S. L. Stanton (Eds.), *Pelvic floor re-education* (1st ed., pp. 7-36). Springer-Verlag London. doi:10.1007/978-1-4471-3569-2_2

44   Yang, C. C., & Bradley, W. E. (1998). Neuroanatomy of the penile portion of the human dorsal nerve of the penis. *British Journal of Urology, 82*(1), 109–113. doi:10.1046/j.1464-410x.1998.00669.x

45   Rojas-Gómez, M., Blanco-Dávila, R., Tobar Roa, V., Gómez González, A., Ortiz Zableh, A., & Ortiz Azuero, A. (2017). Regional anesthesia guided by ultrasound in the pudendal nerve territory. *Colombian Journal of Anesthesiology, 45*(3), 200-209. doi:10.1016/j.rcae.2017.06.007

46   Hitselberger, W., & Witten, R. (1968). Abnormal myelograms in asymptomatic patients. *Journal of Neurosurgery, 28*(3), 204-206. doi:10.3171/jns.1968.28.3.0204

47   Nakashima, H., Yukawa, Y., Suda, K., Yamagata, M., Ueta, T., & Kato, F. (2015). Abnormal findings on magnetic resonance images of the cervical spines in 1211 asymptomatic subjects. *Spine, 40*(6), 392-398. doi:10.1097/brs.0000000000000775

48   Tengan, C. H., Oliveira, A. S., Kiyomto, B. H., Morita, M. P., De Medeiros, J. L., & Gabbai, A. A. (1993). Isolated and painless infraspinatus atrophy in top-level volleyball players. Report of two cases and review of the literature. *Arquivos de Neuro-psiquiatria, 51*(1), 125–129. doi:10.1590/s0004-282x1993000100020

References

49   Moseley, L., & Butler, D. (2017). *Explain pain supercharged.* Noigroup Publications.

50   Nicotra, L., Loram, L., Watkins, L., & Hutchinson, M. (2012). Toll-like receptors in chronic pain. *Experimental Neurology, 234*(2), 316-329. doi:10.1016/j.expneurol.2011.09.038

51   Keller, G. B., & Mrsic-Flogel, T. D. (2018). Predictive processing: A canonical cortical computation. *Neuron, 100*(2), 424–435. doi:10.1016/j.neuron.2018.10.003

52   Flor, H. (2002). Painful memories. *EMBO Reports, 3*(4), 288-291. doi:10.1093/embo-reports/kvf080

53   Moseley, L., & Butler, D. (2017). *Explain pain supercharged.* Noigroup Publications.

54   Penfield, W., & Boldrey, E. (1937). Somatic motor and sensory representation in the cerebral cortex of man as studied by electrical stimulation. *Brain: A Journal of Neurology, 60*(4), 389-443. doi:10.1093/brain/ 60.4.389

55   Catani M. (2017). A little man of some importance. *Brain: A Journal of Neurology, 140*(11), 3055–3061. doi:10.1093/brain/awx270

56   Moseley, L., & Butler, D. (2017). *Explain pain supercharged.* Noigroup Publications.

57   Louw, A., Hilton, S., & Vandyken, C. (2014). *Why pelvic pain hurts: Neuroscience education for patients with pelvic pain.* OPTP.

58   Woolf, C. (2011). Central sensitization: Implications for the diagnosis and treatment of pain. *PAIN, 152*(3 Suppl), S2-S15. doi:10.1016/j.pain.2010.09.030

59   Bordoni, B., & Zanier, E. (2013). Anatomic connections of the diaphragm: influence of respiration on the body system. *Journal of Multidisciplinary Healthcare, 6*, 281–291. doi:10.2147/JMDH.S45443

60   Bordoni, B., & Zanier, E. (2013). Anatomic connections of the diaphragm: influence of respiration on the body system. *Journal of Multidisciplinary Healthcare, 6*, 281–291. doi:10.2147/JMDH.S45443

61   Nair, J., Streeter, K. A., Turner, S. M, Sunshine, M., Bolser, D., Fox, E., Davenport, P. W., & Fuller, D. D. (2019). Anatomy and physiology of phrenic afferent neurons. *Journal of Neurophysiology, 18*(6), 2975–2990. doi:10.1152/jn.00484.2017

62   Wells, R. E., Collier, J., Posey, G., Morgan, F., Auman, T., Strittameter, B., Magalhaes, R., Adler-Neal, A., McHaffie, J. G., & Zeidan, F. (2020). Attention to breath sensations does not engage endogenous opioids to reduce pain. *PAIN, 161*(8), 1884-1893. doi:10.1097/j.pain.0000000000001865

63   Zeidan, F., Adler-Neal, A., Wells, R., Stagnaro, E., May, L., Eisenach, J., McHaffie, J. G., & Coghill, R. C. (2016). Mindfulness-meditation-based pain relief is not mediated by endogenous opioids. *Journal of Neuroscience, 36*(11), 3391-3397. doi:10.1523/jneurosci.4328-15.2016

64   Bordoni, B., & Zanier, E. (2013). Anatomic connections of the diaphragm: influence of respiration on the body system. *Journal of Multidisciplinary Healthcare, 6*, 281–291. doi:10.2147/JMDH.S45443

65   Slater, D., Korakakis, V., O'Sullivan, P., Nolan, D., & O'Sullivan, K. (2019). Sit up straight: Time to re-evaluate. *Journal of Orthopaedic & Sports Physical Therapy, 49*(8), 562–564. doi:10.2519/jospt.2019.0610

References

66   Richards, K. V., Beales, D. J., Smith, A. J., O'Sullivan, P. B., & Straker, L. M. (2016). Neck posture clusters and their association with biopsychosocial factors and neck pain in australian adolescents. *Physical Therapy, 96*(10), 1576-1587. doi:10.2522/ptj.20150660

67   Laird, R., Kent, P., & Keating, J. (2016). How consistent are lordosis, range of movement and lumbo-pelvic rhythm in people with and without back pain?. *BMC Musculoskeletal Disorders, 17*(1), 1-14. doi:10.1186/s12891-016-1250-1

68   Schmidt, H., Bashkuev, M., Weerts, J., Graichen, F., Altenscheidt, J., Maier, C., & Reitmaier, S. (2018). How do we stand? Variations during repeated standing phases of asymptomatic subjects and low back pain patients. *Journal of Biomechanics, 70*, 67-76. doi:10.1016/j.jbiomech.2017.06.016

69   Claus, A. P., Hides, J. A., Moseley, G. L., & Hodges, P. W. (2016). Thoracic and lumbar posture behaviour in sitting tasks and standing: Progressing the biomechanics from observations to measurements. *Applied Ergonomics, 53*, 161-168. doi:10.1016/j.apergo.2015.09.006

70   Garcia, D., Flores, E., Nahuelhual, P., & Solis, F. (2018). Phantom pain in congenital amputees: Myth or reality? *Annals of Physical and Rehabilitation Medicine, 61S*(2018), e118. doi:10.1016/j.rehab.2018.05.258

71   Geneen, L. J., Martin, D. J., Adams, N., Clarke, C., Dunbar, M., Jones, D., McNamee, P., Schofield, P., & Smith, B.H. (2015). Effects of education to facilitate knowledge about chronic pain for adults: a systematic review with meta-analysis. *Systematic Reviews, 4*, 132. doi:10.1186/s13643-015-0120-5.

72   Louw, A., Diener, I., Butler, D. S., & Puentedura, E. J. (2011). The effect of neuroscience education on pain, disability, anxiety, stress in chronic musculoskeletal pain. *Archives of Physical Medicine and Rehabilitation, 92*, 2041-2056. doi:10.1016/j.apmr.2011.07.198

73   Vandyken, C., & Hilton, S. (2017). Physical therapy in the treatment of central pain mechanisms for female sexual function. *Sexual Medicine Reviews, 5*(1), 20-30. doi:10.1016/j.sxmr.2016.06.004

74   Moseley, G., & Butler, D. (2015). Fifteen years of explaining pain: The past, present, and future. *The Journal of Pain, 16*(9), 807-813. doi:10.1016/j.jpain.2015.05.005

75   Raja, S., Carr, D., Cohen, M., Finnerup, N., Flor, H., & Gibson, S. et al. (2020). The revised International Association for the Study of Pain definition of pain. *Pain, Publish Ahead of Print.* doi:10.1097/j.pain.0000000000001939

76   Moseley, L., & Butler, D. (2017). *Explain pain supercharged.* Noigroup Publications.

77   Farmer, M., Chanda, M., Parks, E., Baliki, M., Apkarian, A., & Schaeffer, A. (2011). Brain functional and anatomical changes in chronic prostatitis/chronic pelvic pain syndrome. *The Journal of Urology, 186*(1), 117-124. doi:10.1016/j.juro.2011.03.027

78   Prause, N. (2018). Reward dysregulation in sexual function. In J. Gruber (Ed.), *Oxford handbook of positive emotion and psychopathology.* Oxford University Press.

79   Gogolla, N. (2017). The insular cortex. *Current Biology, 27*(12), R580-R586. doi:10.1016/j.cub.2017.05.010

80   Farmer, M. A., Chanda, M., Parks, E., Baliki, M., Apkarian, A. V., & Schaeffer, A. (2011). Brain functional and anatomical changes in chronic prostatitis/chronic pelvic pain syndrome. *The Journal of Urology, 186*(1), 117-124. doi:10.1016/j.juro.2011.03.027

81   Woodworth D., Mayer, E., Leu, K., Ashe-McNalley, C., Naliboff, D., Labus, J. S., Tillisch, K., Kutch, J. J., Farmer, M. A., Apkarian, A. V., Johnson, K. A., Mackey, S. C., Ness, T. J., Landis, R. J., Deutsch, G., Harris, R. E., Clauw, D. J., Mullins, C., Ellingson, B. M., & MAPP Research Network. (2015). Unique microstructural changes in the brain associated with urological chronic pelvic pain syndrome (UCPPS) revealed by diffusion tensor MRI, super-resolution track density imaging, and statistical parameter mapping: A MAPP network neuroimaging study. *PLOS ONE, 10*(10): e0140250. doi:10.1371/journal. pone.0140250

82   Huang, L., Kutch, J. J., Ellingson, B. M., Martucci, K. T., Harris, R. E., Clauw, D. J., Mackey, S., Mayer, E. A., Schaeffer, A. J., Apkarian A. V., & Farmer, M. A. (2016). Brain white matter changes associated with urological chronic pelvic pain syndrome. *PAIN, 157*(12), 2782-2791. doi:10.1097/j.pain.0000000000000703

83   Wall, P. D., & McMahon, S. B. (1986). The relationship of perceived pain to afferent nerve impulses. *Trends in Neurosciences, 9*(6), 254-255. http://dx.doi.org/10.1016/0166-2236(86)90070-6

84   Brown, T., Chapman, P., Kairiss, E., & Keenan, C. (1988). Long-term synaptic potentiation. *Science, 242*(4879), 724–728. doi:10.1126/science.2903551

85   Malfliet, A., Coppieters, I., Van Wilgen, P., Kregel, J., De Pauw, R., Dolphens, M., & Ickmans, K. (2017). Brain changes associated with cognitive and emotional factors in chronic pain: A systematic review. *European Journal of Pain, 21*(5), 769–786. doi:10.1002/ejp.1003

86   Farmer, M. A., Baliki, M., & Apkarian, A. V. (2012). A dynamic network perspective of chronic pain. *Neuroscience Letters, 520*(2), 197-203. doi:10.1016/j.neulet.2012.05.001

87   Eifert, G. H., & Forsyth, J. P. (2005). *Acceptance and commitment therapy for anxiety disorders: a practitioners treatment guide to using mindfulness, acceptance and values-based behavior change strategies.* New Harbinger.

88   Vandyken, C., & Hilton, S. (2017). Physical therapy in the treatment of central pain mechanisms for female sexual function. *Sexual Medicine Reviews, 5*(1), 20-30. doi:10.1016/j. sxmr.2016.06.004

89   Davidson, R. (2004). What does the prefrontal cortex "do" in affect: perspectives on frontal EEG asymmetry research. *Biological Psychology, 67*(1-2), 219-234. doi:10.1016/j. biopsycho.2004.03.008

90   Jensen, M., Gianas, A., Sherlin, L., & Howe, J. (2015). Pain catastrophizing and EEG-α asymmetry. *The Clinical Journal of Pain, 31*(10), 852-858. doi:10.1097/ajp.0000000000000182

91   Jensen, M. (2015, October 1). Pain catastrophizing and your brain. *Body in Mind.* https://unisa.edu.au/research/Health-Research/Research/Body-in-Mind/

92   Engel, G. L. (1960). A unified concept of health and disease. *Perspectives in Biology and Medicine, 3*(4), 459–485. doi:10.1353/pbm.1960.0020

93   Damasio, A. (2019, February). *About the Psychology of Feeling.* (Keynote presentation presented at The San Diego Pain Summit, San Diego, CA.)

94   Nummenmaa, L., Glerean, E., Hari, R., & Hietanen, J. (2013). Bodily maps of emotions. *Proceedings of the National Academy of Sciences, 111*(2), 646-651. doi:10.1073/pnas.1321664111

95   Damasio, A. (2019, February). *About the Psychology of Feeling.* (Keynote presentation presented at The San Diego Pain Summit, San Diego, CA.)

References

96   Kelly, K. (2013, November 10). Body suspension: why would anyone hang from hooks for fun? *The Guardian*. https://www.theguarian.com/lifeandstyle/2013/nov/10/body-suspension-hang-from-hooks-fun

97   Velnar, T., Bailey, T., & Smrkolj, V. (2009). The wound healing process: An overview of the cellular and molecular mechanisms. *Journal of International Medical Research, 37*(5), 1528–1542. doi:10.1177/147323000903700531

98   Diegelmann, R. F., & Evans, M. C. (2004). Wound healing: an overview of acute, fibrotic and delayed healing. *Frontiers in Bioscience, 9*, 283–289. doi:10.2741/1184

99   Louw, A., Hilton, S., & Vandyken, C. (2014). *Why pelvic pain hurts: Neuroscience education for patients with pelvic pain*. OPTP.

100   Hannibal, K., & Bishop, M. (2014). Chronic stress, cortisol dysfunction, and pain: A psychoneuroendocrine rationale for stress management in pain rehabilitation. *Physical Therapy, 94*(12), 1816-1825. doi:10.2522/ptj.20130597

101   Denson, T. F., Spanovic, M., & Miller, N. (2009). Cognitive appraisals and emotions predict cortisol and immune responses: A meta-analysis of acute laboratory social stressors and emotion inductions. *Psychological Bulletin, 135*(6), 823–853. doi:10.1037/a0016909

102   Denson, T. F., Spanovic, M., & Miller, N. (2009). Cognitive appraisals and emotions predict cortisol and immune responses: A meta-analysis of acute laboratory social stressors and emotion inductions. *Psychological Bulletin, 135*(6), 823–853. doi:10.1037/a0016909

103   Blasini, M., Corsi, N., Klinger, R., & Colloca, L. (2017). Nocebo and pain: An overview of the psychoneurobiological mechanisms. *Pain Reports, 2*(2), e585. doi:10.1097/pr9.0000000000000585

104   Hannibal, K., & Bishop, M. (2014). Chronic stress, cortisol dysfunction, and pain: A psychoneuroendocrine rationale for stress management in pain rehabilitation. *Physical Therapy, 94*(12), 1816-1825. doi:10.2522/ptj.20130597

105   Anderson, R. U., Orenberg, E. K., Morey, A., Chavez, N., & Chan, C. A. (2009). Stress induced hypothalamus-pituitary-adrenal axis responses and disturbances in psychological profiles in men with chronic prostatitis/chronic pelvic pain syndrome. *The Journal of Urology, 182*(5), 2319-2324. doi:10.1016/j.juro.2009.07.042

106   Pierce, A. N., & Christianson, J. A. (2015). Stress and chronic pelvic pain. *Progress in Molecular Biology and Translational Science, 131*, 509-35. doi:10.1016/bs.pmbts.2014.11.009

107   Nickel, J. C., Alexander, R. B., Schaeffer, A. J., Landis, J. R., Knauss, J. S., Propert, K. J., & Chronic Prostatitis Collaborative Research Network Study Group (2003). Leukocytes and bacteria in men with chronic prostatitis/chronic pelvic pain syndrome compared to asymptomatic controls. *The Journal of Urology, 170*(3), 818–822. doi:10.1097/01.ju.0000082252.49374.e9

108   Van der Velde, J., & Everaerd, W. (2001). The relationship between involuntary pelvic floor muscle activity, muscle awareness and experienced threat in women with and without vaginismus. *Behaviour Research and Therapy, 39*(4), 395-408. doi:10.1016/s0005-7967(00)00007-3

109   Michael Phelps. (2020, June 28). In *Wikipedia*. Retrieved from https://en.wikipedia.org/wiki/Michael_Phelps

110   Weir, K. (2018). A growing demand for sport psychologists. *American Psychological Association, 49*(10), 50.

References

111   Dybowski, C., Löwe, B., & Brünahl, C. (2018). Predictors of pain, urinary symptoms and quality of life in patients with chronic pelvic pain syndrome (CPPS): A prospective 12-month follow-up study. *Journal of Psychosomatic Research*, *112*, 99-106. doi:10.1016/j.jpsychores.2018.06.013

112   Wood, N., Qureshi, A., & Mughal, F. (2017). Positioning, telling, and performing a male illness: Chronic prostatitis/chronic pelvic pain syndrome. *British Journal of Health Psychology*, *22*(4), 904-919. doi:10.1111/bjhp.12261

113   Wood, N., Qureshi, A., & Mughal, F. (2017). Positioning, telling, and performing a male illness: Chronic prostatitis/chronic pelvic pain syndrome. *British Journal of Health Psychology*, *22*(4), 904-919. doi:10.1111/bjhp.12261

114   Gyatso, G. K. (2017). *How to transform your life*. Tharpa Publications US.

115   Rankin, L. (2016, September). Can you think yourself well? *TIME Special Edition*, 30-33.

116   Gyatso, G. K. (2015). *How to solve our human problems*. Tharpa Publications US.

117   Van Vliet, C. M., Meulders, A., Vancleef, L., Meyers, E., & Vlaeyen, J. (2019). Changes in pain-related fear and pain when avoidance behavior is no longer effective. *The Journal of Pain*, *00*(0), 1-12. Advance online publication. doi:10.1016/j.jpain.2019.09.002

118   Moseley, G. L., & Arntz, A. (2007). The context of a noxious stimulus affects the pain it evokes. *PAIN*, *133*(1-3), 64–71. doi:10.1016/j.pain.2007.03.002

119   Frankl, V. E. (2006). *Man's search for meaning*. Beacon Press.

120   Rasmussen, H. N., Scheier, M. F., & Greenhouse, J. B. (2009). Optimism and physical health: a meta-analytic review. *Annals of Behavioral Medicine*, *37*(3), 239–256. doi:10.1007/s12160-009-9111-x

121   Hanssen, M. M., Peters, M. L., Vlaeyen, J. W., Meevissen, Y. M., & Vancleef, L. M. (2013). Optimism lowers pain: evidence of the causal status and underlying mechanisms. *PAIN*, *154*(1), 53–58. doi:10.1016/j.pain.2012.08.006

122   Mayer, E. A., Knight, R., Mazmanian, S. K., Cryan, J. F., & Tillisch, K. (2014). Gut microbes and the brain: paradigm shift in neuroscience. *The Journal of Neuroscience*, *34*(46), 15490–15496. doi:10.1523/JNEUROSCI.3299-14.2014

123   Enders, G. (2018). *Gut: The inside story of our body's most underrated organ*. Greystone Books.

124   Enders, G. (2018). *Gut: The inside story of our body's most underrated organ*. Greystone Books.

125   Espinosa-Medina, I., Saha, O., Boismoreau, F., Chettouh, Z., Rossi, F., Richardson, W. D., & Brunet, J. F. (2016). The sacral autonomic outflow is sympathetic. *Science*, *354*(6314), 893–897. doi:10.1126/science.aah5454

126   Horn, J. P. (2018). The sacral autonomic outflow is parasympathetic: Langley got it right. *Clinical Autonomic Research*, *28*(2), 181–185. doi:10.1007/s10286-018-0510-6

127   Rojas-Gómez, M., Blanco-Dávila, R., Tobar Roa, V., Gómez González, A., Ortiz Zableh, A., & Ortiz Azuero, A. (2017). Regional anesthesia guided by ultrasound in the pudendal nerve territory. *Colombian Journal of Anesthesiology*, *45*(3), 200-209. doi:10.1016/j.rcae.2017.06.007

128   Shoskes, D., Wang, H., Polackwich, A., Tucky, B., Altemus, J., & Eng, C. (2016). Analysis of gut microbiome reveals significant differences between men with chronic prostatitis/chronic pelvic pain syndrome and controls. *The Journal of Urology*, *196*(2), 435-441. doi:10.1016/j.juro.2016.02.2959

References

129   Larsen, J. (2017). The immune response to Prevotella bacteria in chronic inflammatory disease. *Immunology, 151*(4), 363-374. doi:10.1111/imm.12760

130   Singh, R. K., Chang, H. W., Yan, D., Lee, K. M., Ucmak, D., Wong, K., Abrouk, M., Farahnik, B., Nakamura, M., Zhu, T. H., Bhutani, T., & Liao, W. (2017). Influence of diet on the gut microbiome and implications for human health. *Journal of Translational Medicine, 15*(73), 1-17. doi:10.1186/s12967-017-1175-y

131   Cresci, G., & Bawden, E. (2015). Gut Microbiome. *Nutrition in Clinical Practice, 30*(6), 734-746. doi:10.1177/0884533615609899

132   Arora, H. C., Eng, C., & Shoskes, D. A. (2017). Gut microbiome and chronic prostatitis/chronic pelvic pain syndrome. *Annals of Translational Medicine, 5*(2), 1-10. doi:10.21037/atm.2016.12.32

133   Enders, G. (2018). *Gut: The inside story of our body's most underrated organ.* Greystone Books.

134   David, L. A., Maurice, C. F., Carmody, R. N., Gootenberg, D. B., Button, J. E., Wolfe, B. E., Ling, A. V., Devlin, A. S., Varma, Y., Fischbach, M. A., Biddinger, S. B., Dutton, R. J., & Turnbaugh, P. J. (2014). Diet rapidly and reproducibly alters the human gut microbiome. *Nature, 505*(7484), 559–563. doi:10.1038/nature12820

135   Myles, I. A. (2014). Fast food fever: reviewing the impacts of the western diet on immunity. *Nutrition Journal, 13*(61), 1-17. doi:10.1186/1475-2891-13-61

136   Minihane, A. M., Vinoy, S., Russell, W. R., Baka, A., Roche, H. M., & Tuohy, K. M., Teeling, J. L., Blaak, E. E., Fenech, M., Vauzour, D., McArdle, H. J., Kremer, B. H. A., Sterkman, L., Vafeiadou, K., Benedetti, M. M., Williams, C. M., & Calder, P. C. (2015). Low-grade inflammation, diet composition and health: current research evidence and its translation. *British Journal of Nutrition, 114*(7), 999-1012. doi:10.1017/s0007114515002093

137   Lenoir, M., Serre, F., Cantin, L., & Ahmed, S.H. (2007). Intense sweetness surpasses cocaine reward. *PLOS ONE, 2*(8), e698. doi:10.1371/journal. pone.0000698.

138   Patnaik, S. S., Laganà, A. S., Vitale, S. G., Butticè, S., Noventa, M., Gizzo, S., Valenti, G., Rapisarda, A. M. C., La Rosa, V. L., Magno, C., Triolo, O., & Dandolu, V. (2017). Etiology, pathophysiology and biomarkers of interstitial cystitis/painful bladder syndrome. *Archives of Gynecology and Obstetrics, 295*(6), 1341–1359. doi:10.1007/s00404-017-4364-2

139   Aeberli, I., Gerber P.A., Hochuli, M., Kohler, S., Haile, S.R., Gouni-Berthold, I., Berthold, H.K., Spinas, G.A., & Berneis, K. (2011). Low to moderate sugar- sweetened beverage consumption impairs glucose and lipid metabolism and promotes inflammation in healthy young men: a randomized controlled trial. *The American Journal of Clinical Nutrition, 94*(2), 479-85. doi:10.3945/ajcn.111.013540

140   Thompson, T., Oram, C., Correll, C. U., Tsermentseli, S., & Stubbs, B. (2017). Analgesic effects of alcohol: A systematic review and meta-analysis of controlled experimental studies in healthy participants. *The Journal of Pain, 18*(5), 499–510. doi:10.1016/j.jpain.2016.11.009

141   Szabo, G., & Saha, B. (2015). Alcohol's effect on host defense. *Alcohol Research: Current Reviews, 37*(2), 159–170.

142   Szabo, G., & Mandrekar, P. (2009). A recent perspective on alcohol, immunity, and host defense. *Alcoholism, Clinical and Experimental Research, 33*(2), 220–232. doi:10.1111/j.1530-0277.2008.00842.x

References

143   Liao, C., Lin, H., & Huang, C. (2016). Chronic prostatitis/chronic pelvic pain syndrome is associated with irritable bowel syndrome: A population-based study. *Scientific Reports, 6*(26939), 1-4. doi:10.1038/srep26939

144   Takano, S., & Sands, D. (2015). Influence of body posture on defecation: a prospective study of "The Thinker" position. *Techniques in Coloproctology, 20*(2), 117-121. doi:10.1007/s10151-015-1402-6

145   Johannsson, H. O., Graf, W., & Påhlman, L. (2005). Bowel habits in hemorrhoid patients and normal subjects. *The American Journal of Gastroenterology, 100*(2), 401–406. doi:10.1111/j.1572-0241.2005.40195.x

146   Sandler, R., & Peery, A. (2019). Rethinking what we know about hemorrhoids. *Clinical Gastroenterology and Hepatology, 17*(1), 8-15. doi:10.1016/j.cgh.2018.03.020

147   Seingsukon, C., Al-dughmi, M., & Stevens, S. (2017). Sleep health promotion: Practical information for physical therapists. *Physical Therapy, 97*(8), 826-836. doi:10.1093/ptj/pzx057

148   Sivertsen, B., Lallukka, T., Petrie, K., Steingrimsdottir, O., Stubhaug, A., & Nielsen, C. (2015). Sleep and pain sensitivity in adults. *PAIN, 156*(8), 1433-1439. doi:10.1097/j.pain.0000000000000131

149   Seingsukon, C., Al-dughmi, M., & Stevens, S. (2017). Sleep health promotion: Practical information for physical therapists. *Physical Therapy, 97*(8), 826-836. doi:10.1093/ptj/pzx057

150   Pollack, J., & Cabane, O.F. (2016, May 11). Your brain has a "delete" button– Here's how to use it. *Fast Company.* www.fastcompany.com/3059634/your-brain-has-a-delete-button-heres-how-to-use-it

151   Hauser, B. (2016, September). Get in the sleep zone. *TIME Special Edition*, 24-27.

152   Seingsukon, C., Al-dughmi, M., & Stevens, S. (2017). Sleep health promotion: Practical information for physical therapists. *Physical Therapy, 97*(8), 826-836. doi:10.1093/ptj/pzx057

153   Kellesarian, S. V., Malignaggi, V. R., Feng, C., & Javed, F. (2018). Association between obstructive sleep apnea and erectile dysfunction: a systematic review and meta-analysis. *International Journal of Impotence Research, 30*(3), 129–140. doi:10.1038/s41443-018-0017-7

154   Seehuus, M., & Pigeon, W. (2018). The sleep and sex survey: Relationships between sexual function and sleep. *Journal of Psychosomatic Research, 112*, 59–65. doi:10.1016/j.jpsychores.2018.07.005

155   LeVay, S., & Baldwin, J. (2012). Men's bodies. In *Human sexuality* (4th ed., pp. 86-116). Sinauer Associates, Inc.

156   Dean, R. C., & Lue, T. F. (2005). Physiology of penile erection and pathophysiology of erectile dysfunction. *The Urologic Clinics of North America, 32*(4), 379–395. doi:10.1016/j.ucl.2005.08.007

157   Travison, T. G., Araujo, A. B., O'Donnell, A. B., Kupelian, V., & McKinlay, J. B. (2007). A population-level decline in serum testosterone levels in American men. *The Journal of Clinical Endocrinology and Metabolism, 92*(1), 196–202. doi:10.1210/jc.2006-1375

158   Travison, T. G., Araujo, A. B., Kupelian, V., O'Donnell, A. B., & McKinlay, J. B. (2007). The relative contributions of aging, health, and lifestyle factors to serum testosterone decline in men. *The Journal of Clinical Endocrinology and Metabolism, 92*(2), 549–555. doi:10.1210/jc.2006-1859

159 Mulhall, J. P., Trost, L. W., Brannigan, R. E., Kurtz, E. G., Redmon, J. B., Chiles, K. A., Lightner, D. J., Miner, M. M., Murad, H., Nelson, C. J., Platz, E. A., Ramanathan, L. V., & Lewis, R. W. (2018). Evaluation and management of testosterone deficiency: AUA guideline. *The Journal of Urology, 200*(2), 423–432. doi:10.1016/j.juro.2018.03.115

160 Lee, J. H., & Lee, S. W. (2016). Testosterone and chronic prostatitis/chronic pelvic pain syndrome: A propensity score-matched analysis. *The Journal of Sexual Medicine, 13*(7), 1047-1055. doi:10.1016/j.jsxm.2016.04.070

161 Marshall, L. (2018, November 14). Pain can be a self fulfilling prophecy. *Neuroscience News.* http://neurosciencenews.com/pain-stimuli-expectation-10193/

162 Jepma, M., Koban, L., van Doorn, J., Jones, M., & Wager, T. (2018). Behavioural and neural evidence for self-reinforcing expectancy effects on pain. *Nature Human Behaviour, 2*(11), 838-855. doi:10.1038/s41562-018-0455-8

163 Atlas, L. Y., & Wager, T. D. (2012). How expectations shape pain. *Neuroscience Letters, 520*(2), 140–148. doi:10.1016/j.neulet.2012.03.039

164 Blasini, M., Corsi, N., Klinger, R., & Colloca, L. (2017). Nocebo and pain: An overview of the psychoneurobiological mechanisms. *Pain Reports, 2*(2), e585. doi:10.1097/pr9.0000000000000585

165 Finniss, D., Kaptchuk, T., Miller, F., & Benedetti, F. (2010). Biological, clinical, and ethical advances of placebo effects. *The Lancet, 375*(9715), 686-695. doi:10.1016/s0140-6736(09)61706-2

166 Benedetti, F., Thoen, W., Blanchard, C., Vighetti, S., & Arduino, C. (2013). Pain as a reward: Changing the meaning of pain from negative to positive co-activates opioid and cannabinoid systems. *PAIN, 154*, 3611-367. doi:10.1016/j.pain.2012.11.007

167 Benedetti, F. (2016, February). *Placebo and Nocebo: Different Contexts, Different Pains.* (Speaker presentation conducted from the San Diego Pain Summit, United States.)

168 Atlas, L. Y., & Wager, T. D. (2012). How expectations shape pain. *Neuroscience Letters, 520*(2), 140–148. doi:10.1016/j.neulet.2012.03.039

169 Benedetti, F., Thoen, W., Blanchard, C., Vighetti, S., & Arduino, C. (2013). Pain as a reward: Changing the meaning of pain from negative to positive co-activates opioid and cannabinoid systems. *PAIN, 154*, 3611-367. doi:10.1016/j.pain.2012.11.007

170 Gyatso, G. K. (2011). *Modern buddhism: The path of compassion and wisdom – Volume 1* sutra. Tharpa Publications US.

171 Moseley, L., & Butler, D. (2015). *Explain pain handbook protectometer.* Noigroup Publications.

172 Butler D., and Moseley, L. (2014). *Explain pain.* Noigroup Publications.

173 Moseley, L., & Butler, D. (2015). *Explain pain handbook protectometer.* Noigroup Publications.

174 Benedetti, F., Thoen, W., Blanchard, C., Vighetti, S., & Arduino, C. (2013). Pain as a reward: Changing the meaning of pain from negative to positive co-activates opioid and cannabinoid systems. *PAIN, 154*, 3611-367. doi:10.1016/j.pain.2012.11.007

175 Harig, B. (2009, June 14). A year later it's time to reminisce. *ESPN.* https://www.espn.com/golf/usopen09/columns/story?columnist=harig_bob&id=4256164

176 Moseley, L., & Butler, D. (2015). *Explain pain handbook protectometer.* Noigroup Publications.

References

177   Jafari, H., Courtois, I., Van den Bergh, O., Vlaeyen, J., & Van Diest, I. (2017). Pain and respiration: a systematic review. *PAIN, 158*(6), 995–1006. doi:10.1097/j.pain.0000000000000865

178   Mindfulness. (2020). *WordHippo.* https://www.wordhippo.com/what-is/the-meaning-of-the-word/mindfulness.html

179   Dahl, J. C., & Lundgren, T. L. (2006). *Living beyond your pain: Using Acceptance and Commitment Therapy to ease chronic pain.* New Harbinger.

180   Emerson, N. M., Zeidan, F., Lobanov, O. V., Hadsel, M. S., Martucci, K. T., Quevedo, A. S., Starr, C. J., Nahman-Averbuch, H., Weissman-Fogel, I., Granovsku, Y., Yarnitsku, D., & Coghill, R. C. (2014). Pain sensitivity is inversely related to regional grey matter density in the brain. *PAIN, 155*(3), 566–573. doi:10.1016/j.pain.2013.12.004

181   Moseley, L., & Butler, D. (2017). *Explain pain supercharged.* Noigroup Publications.

182   Clark, A. (2013). Whatever next? Predictive brains, situated agents, and the future of cognitive science. *Behavioral and Brain Sciences, 36*(3), 181-204. doi:10.1017/s0140525x12000477

183   Sharpe, L. (2019). To focus on pain or not to focus? When is the question. *PAIN, 160*(10), 2173-2174.

184   Kan, L., Zhang, J., Yang, Y., & Wang, P. (2016). The effects of yoga on pain, mobility, and quality of life in patients with knee osteoarthritis: A systematic review. *Evidence-Based Complementary and Alternative Medicine, 2016,* 1-10. doi:10.1155/2016/6016532

185   Saxena, R., Gupta, M., Shankar, N., Jain, S., & Saxena, A. (2017). Effects of yogic intervention on pain scores and quality of life in females with chronic pelvic pain. *International Journal of Yoga, 10*(1), 9-15. doi:10.4103/0973-6131.186155

186   Pearson, N., Prosko, S., & Sullivan, M. (2019). *Yoga and science in pain care: Treating the person in pain.* Singing Dragon Publishers.

187   Kong, L. J., Lauche, R., Klose, P., Bu, J. H., Yang, X. C., Guo, C. Q., Dobos, G., & Cheng, Y. (2016). Tai Chi for chronic pain conditions: A systematic review and meta-analysis of randomized controlled trials. *Scientific Reports, 6,* 1-9. doi:10.1038/srep25325

188   Vartiainen, N., Kirveskari, E., Kallio-Laine, K., Kalso, E., & Forss, N. (2009). Cortical reorganization in primary somatosensory cortex in patients with unilateral chronic pain. *The Journal of Pain, 10*(8), 854-859. doi:10.1016/j.jpain.2009.02.006

189   Flor, H., Braun, C., Elbert, T., & Birbaumer, N. (1997). Extensive reorganization of primary somatosensory cortex in chronic back pain patients. *Neuroscience Letters, 224*(1), 5-8. doi:10.1016/s0304-3940(97)13441-3

190   Wolf, L. D., & Davis, M. C. (2014). Loneliness, daily pain, and perceptions of interpersonal events in adults with fibromyalgia. *Health Psychology, 33*(9), 929–937. doi:10.1037/hea0000059

191   Jaremka, L., Fagundes, C., Glaser, R., Bennett, J., Malarkey, W., & Kiecolt-Glaser, J. (2013). Loneliness predicts pain, depression, and fatigue: Understanding the role of immune dysregulation. *Psychoneuroendocrinology, 38*(8), 1310-1317. doi:10.1016/j.psyneuen.2012.11.016

192   Necka, E. A., & Atlas, L. Y. (2018). The role of social and interpersonal factors in placebo analgesia. *International Review of Neurobiology, 138,* 161–179. doi:10.1016/bs.irn.2018.01.006

193   Bowering, K. J., O'Connell, N. E., Tabor, A., Catley, M. J., Leake, H. B., Moseley, G. L., & Stanton, T. R. (2013). The effects of graded motor imagery and its components on chronic pain: A systematic review and meta-analysis. *The Journal of Pain, 14*(1), 3–13. doi:10.1016/j.jpain.2012.09.007

References

194   Decety J. (1996). The neurophysiological basis of motor imagery. *Behavioural Brain Research*, *77*(1-2), 45–52. doi:10.1016/0166-4328(95)00225-1

195   Morton, S. K., Whitehead, J. R., Brinkert, R. H., & Caine, D. J. (2011). Resistance training vs. static stretching: effects on flexibility and strength. *Journal of Strength and Conditioning Research*, *25*(12), 3391–3398. doi:10.1519/JSC.0b013e31821624aa

196   Weppler, C. H., & Magnusson, S. P. (2010). Increasing muscle extensibility: a matter of increasing length or modifying sensation? *Physical Therapy*, *90*(3), 438–449. doi:10.2522/ptj.20090012

197   Kjaer M. (2004). Role of extracellular matrix in adaptation of tendon and skeletal muscle to mechanical loading. *Physiological Reviews*, *84*(2), 649–698. doi:10.1152/physrev.00031.2003

198   Magnusson, S., Simonsen, E., Dyhre-Poulsen, P., Aagaard, P., Mohr, T., & Kjaer, M. (2007). Viscoelastic stress relaxation during static stretch in human skeletal muscle in the absence of EMG activity. *Scandinavian Journal of Medicine & Science in Sports*, *6*(6), 323-328. doi:10.1111/j.1600-0838.1996.tb00101.x

199   Magnusson, S. P., Simonsen, E. B., Aagaard, P., Gleim, G. W., McHugh, M. P., & Kjaer, M. (1995). Viscoelastic response to repeated static stretching in the human hamstring muscle. *Scandinavian Journal of Medicine & Science in Sports*, *5*(6), 342–347. doi:10.1111/j.1600-0838.1995.tb00056.x

200   Weppler, C. H., & Magnusson, S. P. (2010). Increasing muscle extensibility: a matter of increasing length or modifying sensation? *Physical Therapy*, *90*(3), 438–449. doi:10.2522/ptj.20090012

201   Konrad, A., & Tilp, M. (2014). Increased range of motion after static stretching is not due to changes in muscle and tendon structures. *Clinical Biomechanics*, *29*(6), 636–642. doi:10.1016/j.clinbiomech.2014.04.013

202   Freitas, S. R., Mendes, B., Le Sant, G., Andrade, R. J., Nordez, A., & Milanovic, Z. (2018). Can chronic stretching change the muscle-tendon mechanical properties? A review. *Scandinavian Journal of Medicine & Science in Sports*, *28*(3), 794–806. doi:10.1111/sms.12957

203   Hargrove, T. (2015, October 12). Why do muscles feel tight? *Better Movement*. https://www.bettermovement.org/blog/2015/why-do-muscles-feel-tight

204   Mitchell, J. (2019). *Yoga biomechanics stretching redefined*. Handspring Publishing Limited.

205   Magnusson, S. P. (1998). Passive properties of human skeletal muscle during stretch maneuvers. A review. *Scandinavian Journal of Medicine & Science in Sports*, *8*(2), 65–77. doi:10.1111/j.1600-0838.1998.tb00171.x

206   Krabak, B. J., Laskowski, E. R., Smith, J., Stuart, M. J., & Wong, G. Y. (2001). Neurophysiologic influences on hamstring flexibility: a pilot study. *Clinical Journal of Sport Medicine*, *11*(4), 241–246. doi:10.1097/00042752-200110000-00006

207   Behm, D. G., Blazevich, A. J., Kay, A. D., & McHugh, M. (2016). Acute effects of muscle stretching on physical performance, range of motion, and injury incidence in healthy active individuals: a systematic review. *Applied Physiology, Nutrition, and Metabolism*, *41*(1), 1–11. doi:10.1139/apnm-2015-0235

208   Mitchell, J. (2019). *Yoga biomechanics stretching redefined*. Handspring Publishing Limited.

209   Contracture. (2020). *Etymonline*. https://www.etymonline.com/word/contracture

References

210   Definition of contracture. (2020). *Merriam-webster*. https://www.merriam-webster.com/ dictionary/contracture?utm_campaign=sd&utm_medium=serp&utm_source=jsonld

211   Harvey, L. A., Katalinic, O. M., Herbert, R. D., Moseley, A. M., Lannin, N. A., & Schurr, K. (2017). Stretch for the treatment and prevention of contracture: an abridged republication of a Cochrane systematic review. *Journal of Physiotherapy*, *63*(2), 67–75. doi:10.1016/j. jphys.2017.02.014

212   Harvey, L. A., Katalinic, O. M., Herbert, R. D., Moseley, A. M., Lannin, N. A., & Schurr, K. (2017). Stretch for the treatment and prevention of contracture: an abridged republication of a Cochrane systematic review. *Journal of Physiotherapy*, *63*(2), 67–75. doi:10.1016/j. jphys.2017.02.014

213   Kelly, S., & Beardsley, C. (2016). Specific and cross-over effects of foam rolling on ankle dorsiflexion range of motion. *International Journal of Sports Physical Therapy*, *11*(4), 544–551.

214   Stanton, T., Moseley, G., Wong, A., & Kawchuk, G. (2017). Feeling stiffness in the back: a protective perceptual inference in chronic back pain. *Scientific Reports*, *7*, 1-12. doi:10.1038/ s41598-017-09429-1

215   Mitchell, J. (2019). *Yoga biomechanics stretching redefined*. Handspring Publishing Limited.

216   Jay, G., & Waller, K. (2014). The biology of lubricin: Near frictionless joint motion. *Matrix Biology*, *39*, 17-24. doi:10.1016/j.matbio.2014.08.008

217   Nijs, J., D'Hondt, E., Clarys, P., Deliens, T., Polli, A., Malfliet, A., Coppieters, I., Willaert, W., Yilmaz, S. T., Elma, O., & Ickmans, K. (2019). Lifestyle and chronic pain across the lifespan: An inconvenient truth? *PM&R*, *12*(4), 410-419. doi:10.1002/pmrj.12244

218   Lavie, C. J., Ozemek, C., Carbone, S., Katzmarzyk, P. T., & Blair, S. N. (2019). Sedentary behavior, exercise, and cardiovascular health. *Circulation Research*, *124*(5), 799–815. doi:10.1161/ CIRCRESAHA.118.312669

219   Louw, A., Hilton, S., & Vandyken, C. (2014). *Why pelvic pain hurts: Neuroscience education for patients with pelvic pain*. OPTP.

220   Law, L. F., & Sluka, K. A. (2017). How does physical activity modulate pain? *PAIN*, *158*(3), 369–370. doi:10.1097/j.pain.0000000000000792

221   Geneen, L. J., Moore, R. A., Clarke, C., Martin, D., Colvin, L. A., & Smith, B. H. (2017). Physical activity and exercise for chronic pain in adults: an overview of Cochrane Reviews. *The Cochrane Database of Systematic Reviews*, (4), 1-68. doi:10.1002/14651858.CD011279.pub3

222   Lima, L. V., Abner, T., & Sluka, K. A. (2017). Does exercise increase or decrease pain? Central mechanisms underlying these two phenomena. *The Journal of Physiology*, *595*(13), 4141–4150. doi:10.1113/JP273355

223   Basso, J. C., & Suzuki, W. A. (2017). The effects of acute exercise on mood, cognition, neurophysiology, and neurochemical pathways: A review. *Brain Plasticity*, *2*(2), 127–152. doi:10.3233/BPL-160040

224   Lima, L. V., Abner, T., & Sluka, K. A. (2017). Does exercise increase or decrease pain? Central mechanisms underlying these two phenomena. *The Journal of Physiology*, *595*(13), 4141–4150. doi:10.1113/JP273355

225   Holschneider, D. P., Wang, Z., Guo, Y., Sanford, M. T., Yeh, J., Mao, J. J., Zang, R., & Ro-
       driguez, L. V. (2020). Exercise modulates neuronal activation in the micturition circuit of
       chronically stressed rats: A multidisciplinary approach to the study of urologic chronic pelvic
       pain syndrome (MAPP) research network study. *Physiology & Behavior, 215*(112796), 1-12.
       doi:10.1016/j.physbeh.2019.112796

226   Sanford, M. T., Yeh, J. C., Mao, J. J., Guo, Y., Wang, Z., Zhang, R., Holschneider, D. P., & Rodri-
       guez, L. V. (2020). Voluntary exercise improves voiding function and bladder hyperalgesia in
       an animal model of stress-induced visceral hypersensitivity: A multidisciplinary approach to
       the study of urologic chronic pelvic pain syndrome research network study. *Neurourology and
       Urodynamics, 3*(2), 1-10. doi:10.1002/nau.24270

227   Giubilei, G., Mondaini, N., Minervini, A., Saieva, C., Lapini, A., Serni, S., Bartoletti, R., &
       Carini, M. (2007). Physical activity of men with chronic prostatitis/chronic pelvic pain syn-
       drome not satisfied with conventional treatments-could it represent a valid option? The phys-
       ical activity and male pelvic pain trial: a double-blind, randomized study. *The Journal of Urol-
       ogy, 177*(1), 159–165. doi:10.1016/j.juro.2006.08.107

228   U.S. Department of Health and Human Services. (2018). *Physical activity guidelines for Amer-
       icans* (2nd ed.). U.S. Department of Health and Human Services.

229   Zhang, R., Chomistek, A. K., Dimitrakoff, J. D., Giovannucci, E. L., Willett, W. C., Rosner, B. A.,
       & Wu, K. (2015). Physical activity and chronic prostatitis/chronic pelvic pain syndrome. *Medi-
       cine and Science in Sports and Exercise, 47*(4), 757–764. doi:10.1249/MSS.0000000000000472

230   Geneen, L. J., Moore, R. A., Clarke, C., Martin, D., Colvin, L. A., & Smith, B. H. (2017). Physi-
       cal activity and exercise for chronic pain in adults: an overview of Cochrane Reviews. *The Co-
       chrane Database of Systematic Reviews*, (4), 1-68. doi:10.1002/14651858.CD011279.pub3

231   Malfliet, A., Ickmans, K., Huysmans, E., Coppieters, I., Willaert, W., Bogaert, W. V., Rheel, E.,
       Bilterys, T., Van Wilgen, P., & Nijs, J. (2019). Best evidence rehabilitation for chronic pain part
       3: Low back pain. *Journal of Clinical Medicine, 8*(1063), 1-24. doi:10.3390/jcm8071063

232   Jacobs, D. (2016). *Dermoneuromodulating: Manual treatment for peripheral nerves and espe-
       cially cutaneous nerves.* Tellwell.

233   Goshen, I., Kreisel, T., Ounallah-Saad, H., Renbaum, P., Zalzstein, Y., Ben-Hur, T., Levy-Lahad,
       E., & Yirmiya, R. (2007). A dual role for interleukin-1 in hippocampal-dependent memory pro-
       cesses. *Psychoneuroendocrinology, 32*(8-10), 1106–1115. doi:10.1016/j.psyneuen.2007.09.004

234   Foster, E., Wildner, H., Tudeau, L., Haueter, S., Ralvenius, W. T., Jegen, M., Johannssen, H.,
       Hösli, L., Haenraets, K., Ghanem, A., Conzelmann, K. K., Bösl, M., & Zeilhofer, H. U. (2015).
       Targeted ablation, silencing, and activation establish glycinergic dorsal horn neurons as
       key components of a spinal gate for pain and itch. *Neuron, 85*(6), 1289–1304. doi:10.1016/j.
       neuron.2015.02.028

235   Roudaut, Y., Lonigro, A., Coste, B., Hao, J., Delmas, P., & Crest, M. (2012). Touch sense:
       functional organization and molecular determinants of mechanosensitive receptors. *Chan-
       nels, 6*(4), 234–245. doi:10.4161/chan.22213

236   Behm, D., & Wilke, J. (2019). Do self-myofascial release devices release myofascia? Roll-
       ing mechanisms: A narrative review. *Sports Medicine, 49*(8), 1173-1181. doi:10.1007/
       s40279-019-01149-y

237   Jacobs, D. (2016). *Dermoneuromodulating: Manual treatment for peripheral nerves and espe-
       cially cutaneous nerves.* Tellwell.

References

238   Mitchell, J. (2019). *Yoga biomechanics stretching redefined.* Handspring Publishing Limited.

239   Behm, D., & Wilke, J. (2019). Do self-myofascial release devices release myofascia? Rolling mechanisms: A narrative review. *Sports Medicine, 49*(8), 1173-1181. doi:10.1007/s40279-019-01149-y

240   Kleine-Borgmann, J., Schmidt, K., Hellmann, A., & Bingel, U. (2019). Effects of open-label placebo on pain, functional disability, and spine mobility in patients with chronic back pain: a randomized controlled trial. *PAIN, 160*(12), 2891-2897. doi:10.1097/j.pain.0000000000001683

241   Behm, D., & Wilke, J. (2019). Do self-myofascial release devices release myofascia? Rolling mechanisms: A narrative review. *Sports Medicine, 49*(8), 1173-1181. doi:10.1007/s40279-019-01149-y

242   Denneny, D., Frawley, H. C., Petersen, K., McLoughlin, R., Brook, S., Hassan, S., & Williams, A. C. (2019). Trigger point manual therapy for the treatment of chronic noncancer pain in adults: A systematic review and meta-analysis. *Archives of Physical Medicine and Rehabilitation, 100*(3), 562–577. doi:10.1016/j.apmr.2018.06.019

243   Shah, J. P., Thaker, N., Heimur, J., Aredo, J. V., Sikdar, S., & Gerber, L. (2015). Myofascial trigger points then and now: A historical and scientific perspective. *PM&R, 7*(7), 746–761. doi:10.1016/j.pmrj.2015.01.024

244   Quintner, J. L., & Cohen, M. L. (1994). Referred pain of peripheral nerve origin: an alternative to the "myofascial pain" construct. *The Clinical Journal of Pain, 10*(3), 243–251. doi:10.1097/00002508-199409000-00012

245   Denneny, D., Frawley, H. C., Petersen, K., McLoughlin, R., Brook, S., Hassan, S., & Williams, A. C. (2019). Trigger point manual therapy for the treatment of chronic noncancer pain in adults: A systematic review and meta-analysis. *Archives of Physical Medicine and Rehabilitation, 100*(3), 562–577. doi:10.1016/j.apmr.2018.06.019

246   Quintner, J. L., Bove, G. M., & Cohen, M. L. (2015). A critical evaluation of the trigger point phenomenon. *Rheumatology, 54*(3), 392–399. doi:10.1093/rheumatology/keu471

247   Jacobs, D. (2016). *Dermoneuromodulating: Manual treatment for peripheral nerves and especially cutaneous nerves.* Tellwell.

248   Denneny, D., Frawley, H. C., Petersen, K., McLoughlin, R., Brook, S., Hassan, S., & Williams, A. C. (2019). Trigger point manual therapy for the treatment of chronic noncancer pain in adults: A systematic review and meta-analysis. *Archives of Physical Medicine and Rehabilitation, 100*(3), 562–577. doi:10.1016/j.apmr.2018.06.019

249   Denneny, D., Frawley, H. C., Petersen, K., McLoughlin, R., Brook, S., Hassan, S., & Williams, A. C. (2019). Trigger point manual therapy for the treatment of chronic noncancer pain in adults: A systematic review and meta-analysis. *Archives of Physical Medicine and Rehabilitation, 100*(3), 562–577. doi:10.1016/j.apmr.2018.06.019

250   Shah, J. P., Danoff, J. V., Desai, M. J., Parikh, S., Nakamura, L. Y., Phillips, T. M., & Gerber, L. H. (2008). Biochemicals associated with pain and inflammation are elevated in sites near to and remote from active myofascial trigger points. *Archives of Physical Medicine and Rehabilitation, 89*(1), 16–23. doi:10.1016/j.apmr.2007.10.018

251   Quintner, J. L., Bove, G. M., & Cohen, M. L. (2015). A critical evaluation of the trigger point phenomenon. *Rheumatology, 54*(3), 392–399. doi:10.1093/rheumatology/keu471

References

252   Meister, M. R., Shivakumar, N., Sutcliffe, S., Spitznagle, T., & Lowder, J. L. (2018). Physical examination techniques for the assessment of pelvic floor myofascial pain: a systematic review. *American Journal of Obstetrics and Gynecology, 219*(5), 497.e1–497.e13. doi:10.1016/j.ajog.2018.06.014

253   Quintner, J. L., Bove, G. M., & Cohen, M. L. (2015). A critical evaluation of the trigger point phenomenon. *Rheumatology, 54*(3), 392–399. doi:10.1093/rheumatology/keu471

254   Butler, D. (2000). *The sensitive nervous system.* Noigroup Publications.

255   Shah, J. P., Thaker, N., Heimur, J., Aredo, J. V., Sikdar, S., & Gerber, L. (2015). Myofascial trigger points then and now: A historical and scientific perspective. *PM&R, 7*(7), 746–761. doi:10.1016/j.pmrj.2015.01.024

256   Artus, M., van der Windt, D. A., Jordan, K. P., & Hay, E. M. (2010). Low back pain symptoms show a similar pattern of improvement following a wide range of primary care treatments: a systematic review of randomized clinical trials. *Rheumatology, 49*(12), 2346–2356. doi:10.1093/rheumatology/keq245

257   Moseley, L., & Butler, D. (2017). *Explain pain supercharged.* Noigroup Publications.

258   Denneny, D., Frawley, H. C., Petersen, K., McLoughlin, R., Brook, S., Hassan, S., & Williams, A. C. (2019). Trigger point manual therapy for the treatment of chronic noncancer pain in adults: A systematic review and meta-analysis. *Archives of Physical Medicine and Rehabilitation, 100*(3), 562–577. doi:10.1016/j.apmr.2018.06.019

259   Bishop, M., Bialosky, J., & Alappattu, M. (2020). Riding a tiger. *Journal of Women's Health Physical Therapy, 44*(1), 32-38. doi:10.1097/jwh.0000000000000156

260   Bishop, M., Bialosky, J., & Alappattu, M. (2020). Riding a tiger. *Journal of Women's Health Physical Therapy, 44*(1), 32-38. doi:10.1097/jwh.0000000000000156

261   Artus, M., van der Windt, D. A., Jordan, K. P., & Hay, E. M. (2010). Low back pain symptoms show a similar pattern of improvement following a wide range of primary care treatments: a systematic review of randomized clinical trials. *Rheumatology, 49*(12), 2346–2356. doi:10.1093/rheumatology/keq245

262   Adapted from Dr. Sandy Hilton. *Pain, Science, and Pelvic Health: Manual Therapy and Neurodynamics* (Course in Chicago, 2018.)

263   Proske, U., & Gandevia, S. C. (2012). The proprioceptive senses: their roles in signaling body shape, body position and movement, and muscle force. *Physiological Reviews, 92*(4), 1651–1697. doi:10.1152/physrev.00048.2011

264   Hargrove, T. (2008, September 12). How to improve proprioception? *Better Movement.* www.bettermovement.org/blog/2008/proprioception-the-3-d-map-of-the-body?rq=proprioception

Printed in Great Britain
by Amazon

28608974R00133